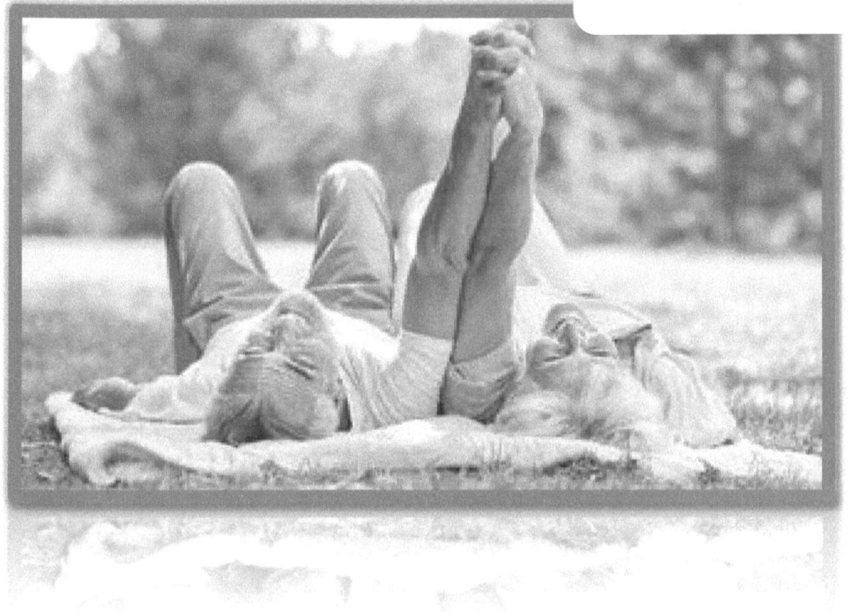

SEX IN YOUR SIXTIES

How to Enjoy Sex Beyond 60
In Fact in Your 50's too!!

By PY Williams

Sex in Your 60's

Contents

IT MUST BE TRUE, ITS IN THE PAPERS

The NHS (National Health Service) in the UK published in their website that 'A third of over-70's report frequent sexual activity.
https://www.nhs.uk/news/older-people/a-third-of-over-70s-report-frequent-sexual-activity/

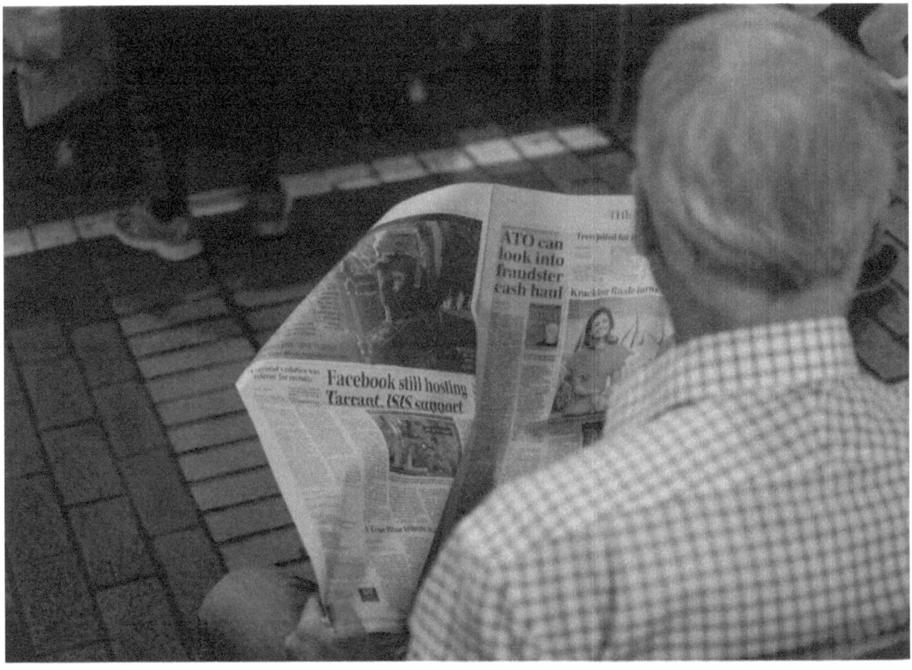

It is based on a study that was carried out by researchers from the University of Manchester, University of Leeds and NatCen Social Research. Funded by the National Institute on Aging and a consortium of UK government departments, so it can be taken far more seriously than tabloid journalism although many national papers did cover the story as they deemed it newsworthy – and it is.

Even though the figure of 'A Third' is published, I believe it is highly likely to be more than a third because there would be a greater degree of privacy and shyness in admitting they were sexually active at their age. It is possible that people, no matter what gender, find it difficult to be honest about this very sensitive topic, even in a confidential questionnaire.

Below: the main findings of the study:

- Data was used from an academic survey of both men and women living in England aged 50 years and older. It is important to note that they were partaking in a study called **The English Longitudinal Study of Ageing (ELSA)**. All the contributors were residing in the community, in private households, not older people in residential care establishments.
- Throughout all the age groups, it was men that reported they had more frequent sexual activity and thought about sex more often than the women participants did. Also, sexually active men reported greater concern over their sexual health and indeed their sexual dissatisfaction than women at all ages.
- It was reported that levels of sexual activity declined as age increased, however a sizable minority of both men and women remain sexually active until their 80's and 90's.
- Poorer health had clear connections with reduced levels of sexual activity and higher numbers of issues with sexual functioning, especially among men.
- It is interesting that the most frequent difficulties reported by sexually active women related to 32% becoming sexually aroused and 27% achieving orgasms whilst with 39% of men reported their main difficulty was erectile function.
- 11% of women reported sexual health concerns, mostly related to their level of sexual desire and 8% related to the frequency of sexual activities.
- 15% of the men had concerns as to their level of sexual desire and 14% reported erectile difficulties.

- The likelihood of men reporting sexual health concerns tended to increase with age in men, but the opposite was seen in women.
- Lesser sexual functioning and disagreements with their partners in relation to the initiation and/or sense of obligation to have sex were associated with greater concerns about and dissatisfaction with overall sex life.

So, according to this study, not only are many older people are still enjoying an active sex-life, older people are very much like every other age group, they have their share of worries and concerns about sex and relationships. It isn't surprising that ageing and health deterioration affects older people's sexual activity.

If we compare older men's concerns with older women's, men reported concerns about getting erections, whilst women worry about the lack of desire.

If you are experiencing problems with your sex life, or simply wish to give it a boost, read on!

A healthy sex life is possible well into your golden years.

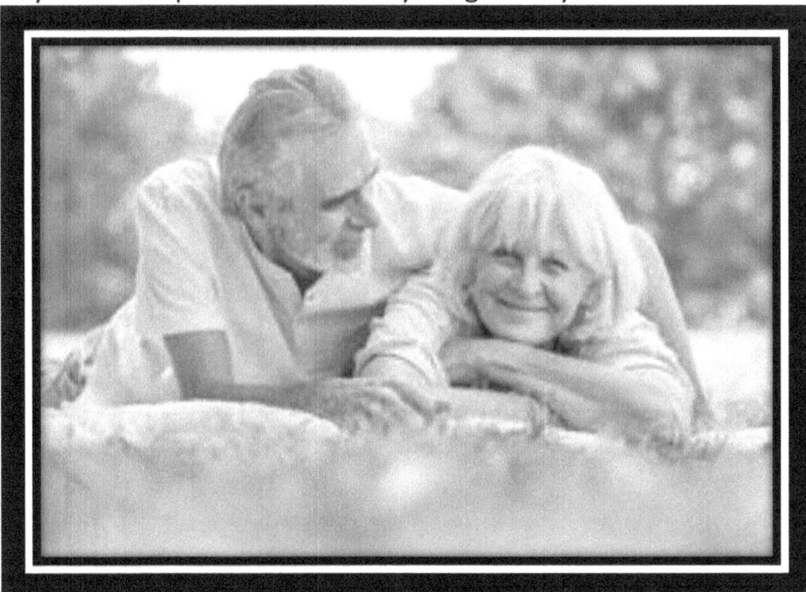

RETIRE FROM WORK YES, BUT NOT FROM YOUR SEX LIFE

Retiring from your job certainly does not mean retiring from an active sex life.

Imagine, that you have 20 years to enjoy retirement.

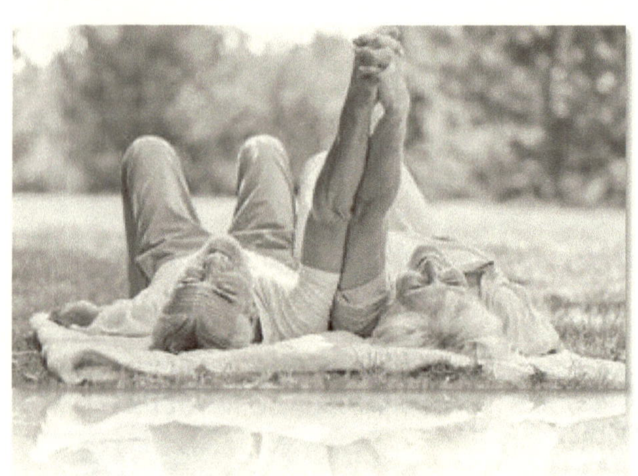

That could be a third of the life you had already lived, the first ten years you were growing up, the second ten years you were probably starting a home and family, just living, getting by and the last twenty years probably working hard, that's your 60 years gone by.

Now you've dearly love to live those 20 years and do some catching up.

Clearly there will be some common health issues, they come naturally at that age, the good news is that there are medical solutions for all, if not of them.

Put aside the natural/normal ailments like vision deterioration and maybe hearing loss because they won't affect your sex life!

Despite the other common ageing issues, whether they are stiffness and aches, or energy levels and concentration, there are so many ways to stay healthy during your retirement. These all contribute in some way to improving or maintain and active sex life.

Exercise

Believe it or not exercise can help with your mood, manage stress, and even increase self-esteem. These are really important issues because they are all an essential part of improving your sex life. Yes, exercise can prevent disease and help improve your blood circulation to the extremities. Better circulation can lead to an improved sexual response in men and women. Exercise doesn't have to be vigorous, you don't need to go to the gym, just a nice brisk walk around the park or even neighborhood, to the shop is a good start. You will see your cognitive function improve and feel better for moving. Apart from helping your sex life, your retirement itself will benefit enormously.

Eat foods that can improve your sex life

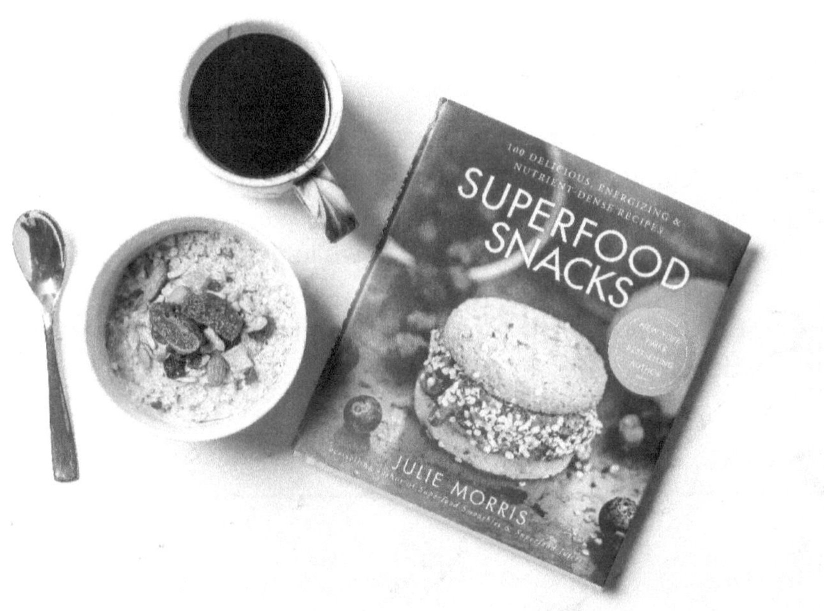

Eating properly is essential anyway, but in terms of eating well to improve your sex life, isn't about aphrodisiacs and myths about oysters. Eating properly promotes energy, it helps reduce the risks of heart disease and works towards getting it pumping properly. Eating the right foods also helps with weight control, which is important as we age, as well as improving our agility in bed and out. Eating the right foods does not have to be complicated and we will cover these later in this eBook

Limit Alcohol Intake

Alcohol and sex have gone together for centuries and may provide some funny memories as well as unforgettable hangovers. Not to mention incidents that are regrettable on many levels.

Over a varied period of time alcohol consumption affects all parts of our body including our brain, heart, immune system, and pancreas, it impairs our vision too.

Like most things in life, moderation is fine, a glass of wine, measure sprits or beer every now and again is fine, but heavy consumption is certainly not recommended.

Alcohol is in fact a depressant, yet we consume it to enjoy the taste and affects. Consuming it heavily can dampen mood, whilst it might appear to increase sexual desire, but it often makes it very difficult for a man to achieve erections or reach an orgasm while under the influence.

The truth is, overdoing the booze is a common cause of erectile dysfunction.

SO, WHAT HAPPENED TO OUR SEX LIFE?

Older people still enjoy and indeed desire sex just as much as younger people, but age is often used as a barrier or excuse, well that stops here, right now.

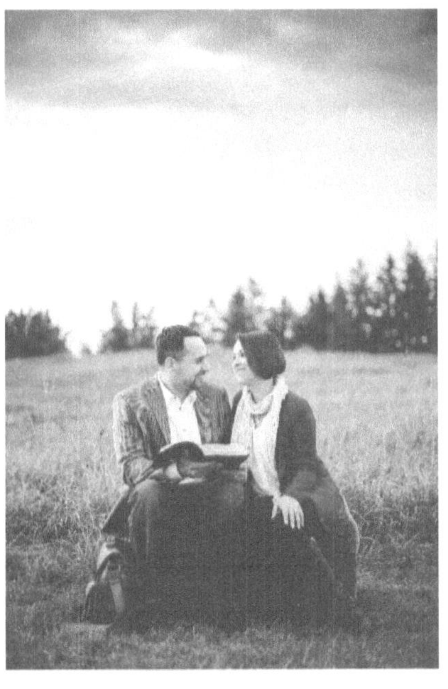

It is fair to say that most hindrances or obstacles that prevent us from enjoying a rewarding sex life after 50 or 60 are generally social and medical issues such as erectile dysfunction, dryness and an inability to achieve an orgasm.

In today's modern world with advances in medicine and accessible therapy or activity there is no reason that they should be a barrier.

Where do these barriers come from? There are so many people over the age of fifty or sixty, indeed seventy that are having a rewarding sex life. Then suddenly, something triggers, and the joy of sex starts to decline.

Often these triggers come from highly trusted sources such as doctors or well-meaning family members, carers/caregivers and friends.

Some take on the stance that when we reach a certain age, we automatically become the asexual oldie that should just do bingo and dominos.

Could the younger generation of doctors jump to the conclusion that their older patients are electively sexually inactive?

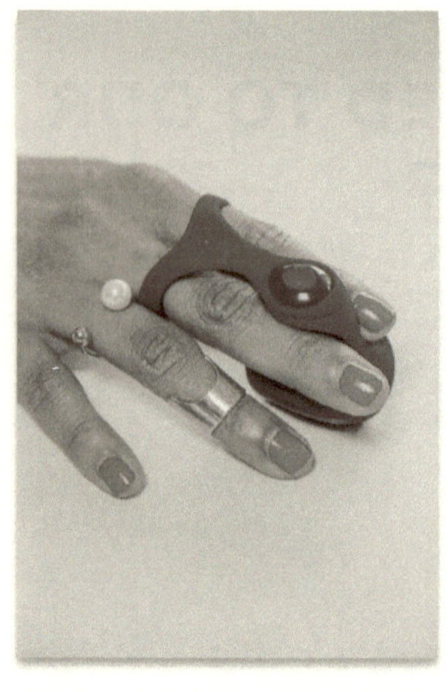

Maybe they are not buying into the myth that sex stops at a certain age but trying to save themselves from a potentially embarrassing conversation with you about your sex life? Especially if they are close to you and your family even in a professional capacity.

Not all doctors are described as above, many are switched on and up to date and not only capable of helping you but they are happy to help you through these times so embrace their skills.

The truth is, if your body, or part of it isn't functioning as it used to, you are entitled to bring the subject up with your doctor. It is vitally important to talk with those who help you in your daily life.

It isn't all about body parts that are not working properly even though some can be fixed with an adjustment or two as you will learn in this eBook.

Let's be honest, a major setback in maintaining a healthy sex life could quite simply the lack of a partner through some form of separation, divorce and bereavement.

Many people over fifty and sixty find themselves widowed or separated and possibly, still with many years of healthy, active life ahead of them.

Gone are the days of widows and widowers bringing abstinence from sex in memory of their spouse. It isn't totally extinct, but the ethos probably ceased being commonplace during the reign of Queen Victory and she set a standard.

There could well be a few readers who are old fashioned and have chosen to abstain from sex out of respect. In the passing of time many accept that the last thing their deceased spouse would really want after their passing is to leave their loved one forever unhappy and unfulfilled. They come to terms with the belief that the real way to truly honour the memory of their departed is to make the most out of the years ahead and live life to the full.

There are hundreds, if not thousands of celebrities who can be considered 'sex symbols. Without creating a huge list, here's a few that come to mind and yes, it is a matter of taste and personal opinion.

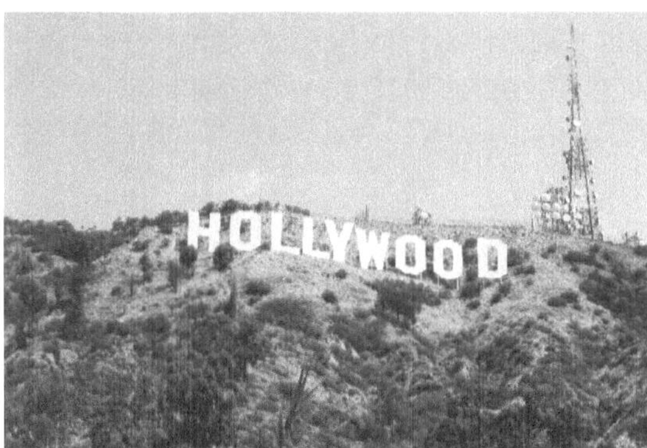

Liam Neeson
Michelle Pfeiffer
Clint Eastwood
Jamie Lee Curtis
Daniel Day-Lewis
George Clooney
Elizabeth Hurley

Most over 60's don't need reminding that it is still very possible to be attractive, indeed it is often the case that people peak at a certain age, they look elegant, feel sexy and have the desire to live healthy and active sex life.

We still encounter the younger people, the stereotypes that in their minds over 50's and 60's are 'over the hill' but, they are still struggling up, we're taking it easy coming down!
Don't let it get to you, people can ignorant and indeed there are those who can be inattentive to the sexual needs of those older, but they have a lot to learn.

It's not even younger people, many who are approaching the 60's are drawn into the endless discouragement of some media bias and people who don't have the facts, they get the 'drip-drip' so-called banter from friends and family too. Soon they simply give up on maintaining a healthy sex life.

Let's get down to the basics, sex begins with desire and the very first step to embarking upon a rewarding sex life is acknowledgement. It is important that you acknowledge yourself as an attractive, desirable individual.

It isn't just about making an effort, although that is important, it is also about disregarding any discouraging remarks and banter that it is aimed at you.

The term 'mutton dressed as lamb' has been bandied about for years and is based on a 40 something dressed as a 20 something.

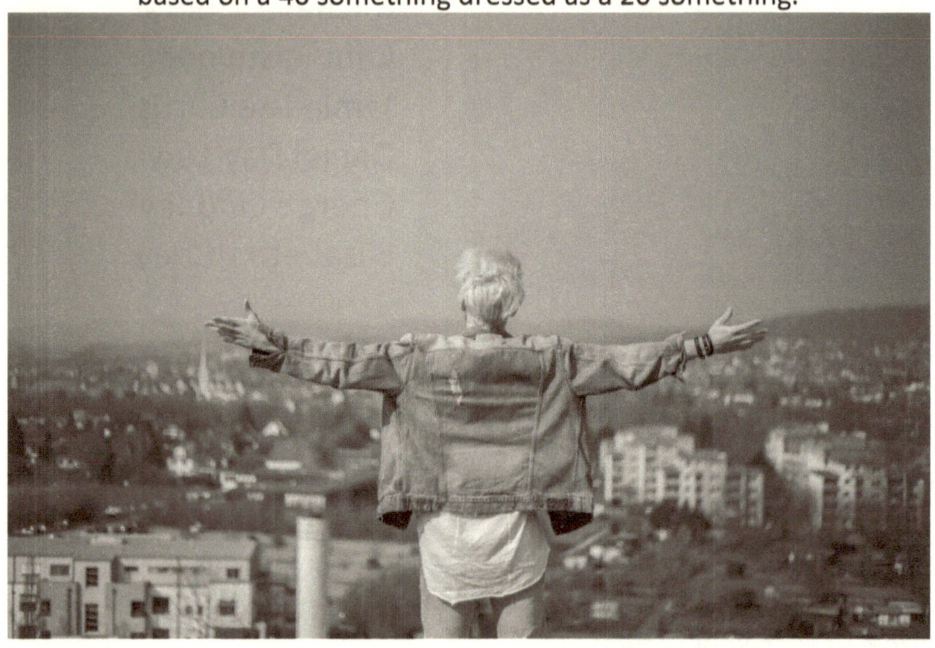

Nowadays people in their 50's, 60's and 70's can shop in the same stores as

people in their 40's – it is socially acceptable and indeed there are people in their 40's who like the look of the more smarter, elegant look.

If you read gossip rags, bitchy TV shows and celebrity style magazines that make you angry or feel uncomfortable with your own image, stop reading and watching them, it cannot be simpler.

Sex in your 60'sIf the people who you associate with make negative comments and indicate that they find it ridiculous for you to still consider looking for a sex partner at your age, just tell them that it is none of their business and their comments are offensive, it doesn't matter what they think. If they make you feel uncomfortable with yourself and indeed their company ditch them.

It's about self-esteem and if you don't feel desirable, how can you be desired? Self-confidence comes from feeling good, feeling good comes from looking good.

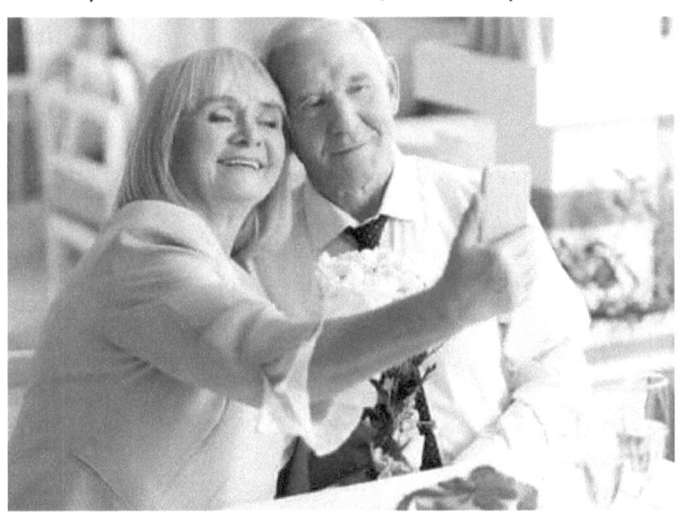

Even enjoying a healthy sex life boosts your self-esteem and makes you feel good, when you feel good, you ooze self-confidence and attract people. All of a sudden people start a conversation with you, at the checkout, in a carpark, post office, bus stop – people out of the blue instigating a chat! Get used to it.

Yes, maintaining a healthy sex life after the age of fifty or sixty maybe hard work, eating properly and keeping fit might seem like an uphill battle, but it is worth it. Disregard those stumbling blocks and break through the obstacles, don't give up on an extremely rewarding part of what it is natural.

Look at a healthy sex life as a personal declaration that you're not nearly over with it all yet, and your best years are still ahead of you. Tell the world that you reduce to sit around for the rest of your life waiting to kick the bucket.

SEX IN TODAY'S WORLD

It seems that in the 2020's sex on TV and cinema is common place but, even advertisements can be sexy but if we rewind a decade at a time, sex and indeed nudity was quite scarce.

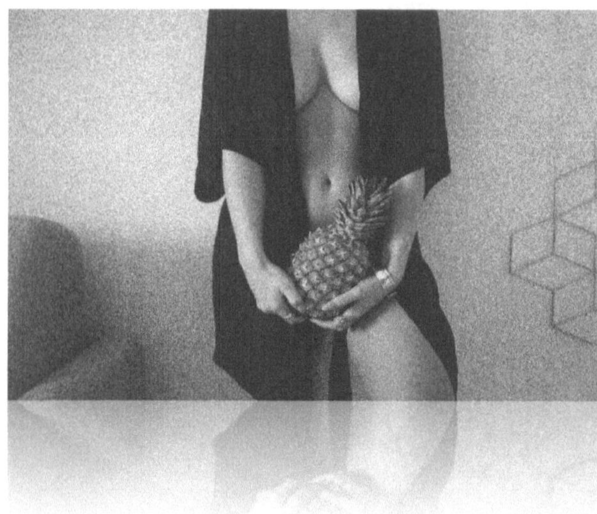

The Kiss (1896) was the first kiss on film but Hollywood did not show nudity onscreen for a very long time, we were guarded from it. There were some movies way back in the silent era that included fully naked bodies, however, from 1934 to 1968, strict censorship monitored every studio film closely for explicit content, even to the point that they flagged costumes that they considered too revealing or indeed shots that were too close for comfort. By the early 1960s, a few up and coming movie stars were brave enough to test the nude taboo.

Enter Marilyn Monroe, she appeared in two nude scenes, 1961 *The Misfits* and1962 *Something's Gotta Give* although neither really made it into the cinemas in one piece.

Very few of us can say we have never heard of 'Fifty Shades of Grey', before that may be 'Lady Chatterley's Lover?

Quite apparently, many people before the 'naughty nineties' were very reluctant or strictly adverse to openly discussing sex. In fact, there is a big contradiction, we might not have discussed sex but wasn't averse to sending a smutty postcard!

Life has changed or I should say 'society has changed' and we are now witnessing a whole range of alternative sexual lifestyles are becoming accepted in our society.

The term 'for better or for worse' was part of a marriage vow between husband and wife, as in male and female. Today, it is generally and legally accepted in same-sex marriages, despite the most prudish minority who still frown upon and indeed cast judgment even upon consenting adults doing whatever they please in the privacy of their own homes.

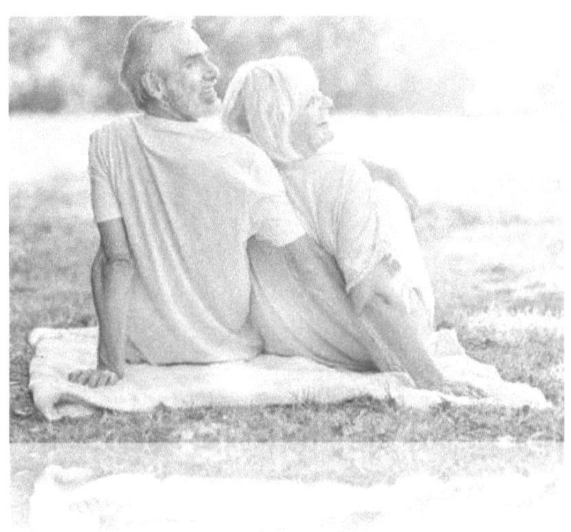

One of today's most crucial developments in this new era of change has been wider acceptance of the sexual needs of women. This is far spread throughout the world because in the recent past, in many western sub-cultures, women were obliged to remain in the background, tradition dictated that they be indirect and play hard to get, they had to skirt around the subject of sex,.

Today women can safely and proudly talk about sex in a direct manner with anyone they trusted and without fear of being called a slut with loose morals.

Let's take a scenario where a couple are on a date and future relationships look promising. Sex is on the cards if things go well. How are they going to learn of each other sexual history, let alone consider the risks of sexually transmitted diseases and other health issues if they don't talk about them?

Open communication is important. Today it is accepted that women should be able to discuss openly about sex, especially with their partners or potential partners. These talks promote a much healthier, more productive, and more efficient relationship. Both partners must be able to communicate with the utmost honesty in terms of what their needs really are.

Do you remember Dr. Ruth?

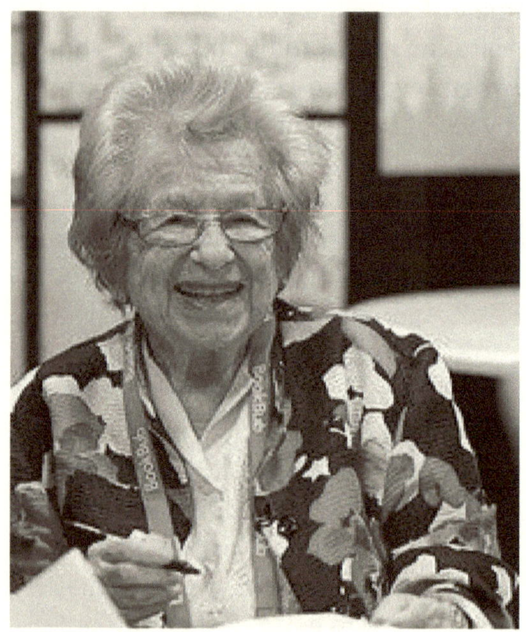

Ruth Westheimer, an American sex therapist, big media personality in her day. She was an author, radio, television talk show host, and Holocaust survivor. Her media career began in 1980 with the radio show **Sexually Speaking**, which continued until 1990.

She was mainly famous for encouraging people to talk openly about sex with their friends, with their doctors and with their partners.

More importantly Dr. Ruth focused on the health aspects of sex, including measures of safe sex practice, and on the personal benefits of maintaining an active sex life.

The message here, about sex in today's world is simply this: Do not be afraid to ask a question. Be perfectly frank with others, if your doctor or partner does have a tendency to withdraw at the idea of open, no holds barred discussions on sex, that really is their problem, and they certainly have to get over it.

SEX AND HEALTH

There are many facets to good, regular sex. Clearly, the sensual and emotional pleasure along with the fulfillment derived from the actual act of sex, but there is more. Proper clinical studies have reported that there are many health benefits gained from having sex on a regular basis.
Back in 1997 a study published in the British Medical Journal reported that men who abstain from sex have twice the mortality rate of men who remained sexually active.

Below is just a small list of these benefits, there are many more.

- **Reduced risk of heart disease**
  Clinical research findings released in 2001 showed results that men who had sex about three times a week cut their risk for stroke and heart attack by half.

  Sexual activity does help to maintain good levels of hormones, such as estrogen and testosterone. When these hormones are out of balance, you could develop conditions such as heart disease and osteoporosis. Have sex and help protect your heart, more sex the better. One study showed that men who had sex at least 2 times a week were 50% less likely to die of heart disease than their less sexually active peers.

- **Physical fitness**
  Just like all other types of physical activity, sex really does burn calories too! We can break this down. If you sit and watch T.V you will burn about one calorie per minute. Having sex can increase your heart rate as well as utilise various muscle groups, it will burn about 5 calories per minute (about the same number of calories burned by

enjoying an active, healthy sex life is a nice way to get some extra physical activity. Some wise person did say that the bed was the greatest exercise machine ever invented! Rigorous sex and low impact exercise are often recommended as a great way to stay in shape. A bonus is that the pulse rate more than doubles, it increases from an average of seventy beats per minute to an average of one hundred and fifty beats per minute when a person is sexually aroused. More bonuses… The muscle contractions work much of the body during sex, along with the pelvis, thighs, arms, chest, neck and buttocks. An activity that tones and strengthens the muscles. Sex also increases a person's testosterone levels, in both men and women, this leads to a stronger musculoskeletal system, so, all in all, sex is an excellent preventative measure against osteoporosis.

- **Reduced depression and Stress**
  Sex really is an excellent stress reliever. This is because the intimate sensual touching, hugging, and emotional attachment stimulates the release of "feel good" hormones and chemicals that promote bonding and calmness. Sexual arousal also releases substances that stimulate the reward and pleasure system in the brain. It can help relieve anxiety and boost overall health.
  In a 2002 clinical study of three hundred women, it was recorded that, amongst sexually active women whose partners did not use condoms, they were generally less prone to depression than the others. One theory is that it has to do with prostaglandin, a hormone exists only in semen. When the semen is absorbed along the female genital tract, it is suspected to have a positive effect on the woman's hormones.

- **Better immune system**
  Clinical research from the Wilkes University in Pennsylvania shows that having sex at least once or twice a week boosts your levels of immunoglobulin A, this is an antibody that supports the immune system. So, getting colds or the flu far less often.

Could sex help you live longer? Well, it may be that having more sex could really help. In a study lasting ten years, involving over 1,000 middle-aged men, the subjects who achieved the most orgasms had half the death rate compared with those who did not ejaculate frequently

- **Lower blood pressure**
  Sex can help lower blood pressure. There are many clinical studies that document a solid link between intercourse, this means proper intercourse and not just masturbation to lower systolic blood pressure. Systolic is the first number on a blood pressure test. Sex sessions do not replace blood-pressure lowering drugs to control high blood pressure.

- **Lessen pain**
  Sexual stimulation and this time it includes masturbation with orgasm can help keep lessen pain. These two activities can reduce pain sensation and increase your pain threshold. Orgasms release hormones that help block pain signals. It has been reported that some women who masturbation can reduce symptoms of menstrual cramps, arthritis, and even headache.

- **Reduce prostate cancer**
  There are health benefits of sex that are male-specific. One clinical study recorded that men who achieved ejaculations at a frequency of over 21 times a month were less likely to develop prostate cancer than men who achieved fewer ejaculations. There was no difference if the ejaculations were through intercourse, masturbation, or even wet dreams. It is important to note that there is far more to prostate cancer risk than the frequency of ejaculations, but the findings of the study are interesting.

- **Look younger**
  You can spend a fortune on surgery and indeed anti-aging creams, but good old-fashioned sex keeps you looking younger too. It is true, regular sex stimulates the release of estrogen and testosterone.

interesting study, participants were viewed through a one-way mirror and judges were asked to guess their ages. Those who had participated in sex at least 4 times per week were perceived to be 7 to 12 years younger than their real age.

- **Better bladder control**
Stemming the flow of urine works the same set of muscles that we put to work during sex, in turn regular intercourse can strengthen these muscles and improve bladder control.

  Urinary incontinence affects about a third of the female population at some point in their life. Having regular orgasms helps to work women's' pelvic floor muscles, it strengthens and tones them. Orgasms activate exactly the same set of muscles that women use when doing Kegel exercises. So having stronger pelvic muscles means there's less risk of those little but embarrassing accidents and urine leaks.

  How to do Kegel Exercises

  1. Make sure your bladder is empty, then sit or lie down.
  2. Tighten your **pelvic floor** muscles. Hold tight and count 3 to 5 seconds.
  3. Relax the muscles and count 3 to 5 seconds.
  4. Repeat 10 times, 3 times a day (morning, afternoon, and night).

Wouldn't you rather have orgasms?

The above-mentioned examples are just a few of the health benefits of sex. There are many studies that have also reported that subjects who have sex regularly to have better teeth. Perhaps the best health advice a person can receive is simply to have sex regularly.

Sex in Your 60's

Needless to say, the human body has to be kept healthy and regular exercise with proper nutrition is important for us all to experience a fulfilling sex life.

The reality is many of the most common problems relating to sex have been connected directly to poor health and lack of proper nutrition.

So, a lack of sex drive or no interest in sex, impotency, premature climax, sterility, fatigue and a whole host of other problems have been linked directly to poor diets and inactive lifestyles.

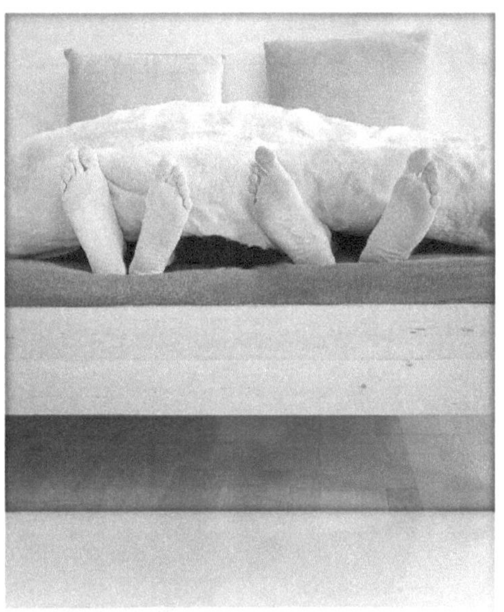

By virtue of the fact that you are reading this eBook indicates that sex plays a major part in your life, or you would certainly like it to.

However, sex is only one part of life, it is a cog and a person's entire lifestyle, all the other cogs must be maintained sufficiently in order for a sex life to be rewarding.

FOODS THAT CAN IMPROVE SEX.

Sex is meant to be enjoyed and not finished far too quickly.

On the other hand, you don't have to go all night just to please your partner.

A study in the _Journal of Sexual Medicine_ reported that the average time couples spend having sexual intercourse ranges from three to thirteen minutes, that's a pretty big ten minute difference.

It isn't the only research; others have revealed that most females, when they want sex, would like good quality sex to last between 15 and 25 minutes. They don't want it to go on for hours, nor do they want it to be over in a couple of minutes.

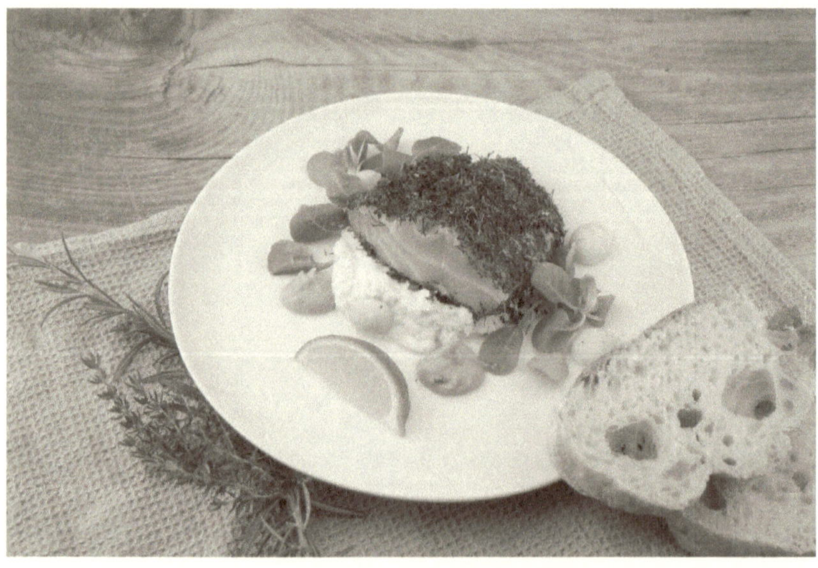

Are there foods that really will help boost your staying power?
The short answer is "yes"! and here is a pretty extensive list for you to feast on.

- **Apples**. We've all chanted "An apple a day keeps the doctor away" at some time in our lives. Little did we know that apples may also help with our staying power and extend our sexual stamina. Apples have high levels of an antioxidant flavonoid called quercetin, it is also found in many other foods, such as onions, green tea, apples, berries, Ginkgo biloba, St. John's wort, and more, People use quercetin as a medicine. Quercetin has been found to play an important role in improving endurance, including extending your time in sexual activity. Quercetin also helps to prevent the release of cortisone, this causes muscle breakdown, so you will be able to enjoy sex longer without experiencing premature fatigue.

- **Asparagus**. Another B vitamin that helps maintain levels of oxygen in our blood and produces healthy cells. Asparagus is known to help our focus, energy, and alertness. It is one of the best sources of folate in our diets—just a handful of spears will provide you with a third of your recommended daily intake.

- **Avocado** helps with sexual stamina. If you have anxiety issues especially about sex, this could be elevating your stress levels too, as a result, your libido plummets and gets in the way of a longer, better sex. In addition, a lack of B-vitamins could also be making your stress worse, according to a *Nutrition Journal* study. There is an easy solution. Have some guacamole! Avocados are rich in stress-relieving B vitamins, as well as a great source of monounsaturated fat, proven to help blood flow to the entire body, obviously including the penis. Read the *Journal of Hypertension* study.

- **Bananas**. Full of simple carbs to provide extra energy and potassium to help you with your stamina. Bananas have a muscle-relaxing mineral that helps to prevent cramps and muscle spasms which really could put the dampeners on sex. The Ameri can boost sexual performance by managing better blood flow to crucial parts of the body, including genitals.

- **Basil** improves circulation and blood flow improves libido. Basil also has a sense of warming on the body that can enhance arousal.

- **Beans and Legumes**. It is well documented that beans, peas, and lentils contain zinc, very important for adrenal function.

- **Beef** helps boost and maintain libido, niacin (Vitamin B3). A study in the _Journal of Sexual Medicine_ reported that men suffering from impotence and took a niacin supplement reported significant improvements in their sex-life more than men who took a placebo. We're not talking great big lumps of steak here, just 3 ounces of good quality beef will serve up 30 percent of the daily recommended intake.

- **Beetroots**. It contains a high level of boron, a mineral boron that boosts the production of sexual hormones and , beetroot juice could increase your libido, Drinking beetroot juice can also help women's bodies to metabolise and use oestrogen it also increases testosterone levels in men.

- **Broccoli**, just like sprouts are usually ignored by men, but that certainly is their loss because broccoli contains indole-3-carbinol also known as I3C and is widely sold as a sex improvement enhancer.

   It can reduce estrogen levels in men, giving their libido a much-needed boost.

- **Chia seeds** also rich in protein, fibre, iron, zinc (which is for testosterone), all help to boost stamina and circulation. They also help sensitize the nerve endings for an added sensory experience. .

- **Chili Peppers**. Add some serrano peppers to a stir fry, jalapenos to guacamole, or cayenne pepper to your eggs. Each of these peppers contain a significant amount of capsaicin, this is natural chemical that puts the heat into Tabasco sauce. It releases certain chemicals that increase heart rate.

Why chili? Why increase the heart rate? The sensation of a faster pulse is the same as signs of arousal, and in turn releases feel-good endorphins. So, chili peppers won't just boost your metabolism, they may even put you in the mood for passion as well as increasing your staying power.

- **Dark chocolate**. Did you know that stress and performance anxiety account for up to 20 percent of all erection problems? Could you be letting your partner down or indeed letting yourself down because you feel down in the dumps? We know chocolate seems to be the 'go to' treat when things aren't working out and there is some logic in it because eating certain foods can counteract stress. Dark chocolate being one of them. According to research, cacao increases our levels of serotine, the mood-boosting hormone. Cacao is a pure form of chocolate that comes very close to the raw and natural state in which it is harvested.

  A 30-day trial where subjects who consumed a daily chocolate drink reported feeling much calmer and soother than participants who didn't sip the chocolate beverage.

  A study in the *Journal of Sex Medicine* equally found that sexual desire and sexual pleasure increased in women after eating some dark chocolate.

- **Flax seed** another superfood but this one increases libido in women. Flaxseeds contain phytoestrogens that act very similarly to female hormones that are linked to a healthy sex life. These are estrogen-like chemicals have antiviral, antibacterial, and anticancer properties.

  Flax can be beneficial for women who have low estrogen levels, such improve cardiovascular health, a plus for libido. Also, L-arginine. This amino acid can boost blood flow and keep sperm healthy.

- **Garlic**, it's been used as far back as the ancient Egyptians to boost their stamina. A *Journal of Nutrition* study reported that consuming garlic extract can help prevent the formation of those fatty deposits inside arterial walls including the arteries leading to the penis, too. By maintaining a healthy heart, erections can be stronger so add some garlic to your food. The downside is that garlic will not make your breath smell sexy so remember the mint!

- **Ginger**. Another food that can improve your sex life. It aids blood flow and and according to a study in the *International Journal of Cardiology*, just consuming one teaspoon of the ginger a few times a week is enough to reap the benefits.

- **Goji Berries,** a superfood known to increase libido. They are exotic berries although widely available now and are said to boost energy levels. They may also increase testosterone production which is a win-win for both men and women in their love lives.

- **Nutmeg** is a well-known spice used in Indian medicine to boost libido and some animal clinical research suggests that high doses of nutmeg may enhance libido and sexual performance. Only grate a tiny amount into foods though. A little goes a long way.

- **Nuts.** Pistachios, peanuts, and walnuts contain the amino acid L-arginine, you'll see this cropping up here quite often, it is one of the building blocks of nitric oxide, not as sinister as it sounds though. It is a naturally occurring gas that helps men maintain erections. Those nuts mentioned above are also high in magnesium to boost energy and endurance. The added bonus is that these nuts can help reduce cholesterol levels, according to a study Nutrition, Metabolism and Cardiovascular Diseases. So, the less cholesterol we host, the better it is for blood to circulate throughout our body and equally as important down towards our penis, this can help preserve a firm erection for a longer time..

- **Oats**. Just one cup of oats contain 688 milligrams of L-arginine, the amino acid we mentioned in water melon that is used to treat erectile dysfunction.

- **Olive Oil** and indeed following the Mediterranean diet may well help those with sexual dysfunction issues because it is known as a 'healthy fat' and one of the foods that can increase libido in men.

   The heart too benefits because olive oil helps with cardiovascular health and in turn promotes healthy blood vessels which are necessary in maintaining an erection and sustained blood flow.

- **Pomegranate Juice**. A study published in the *International Journal of Impotence Research* reported that pomegranate juice being rich in antioxidants that support flow of blood can help improve erectile dysfunction.

- **Pumpkin seeds** are nutritional superfoods with sources of zinc and magnesium proven to boost testosterone levels. According to an *International Journal of Endocrinology* study. The magnesium decreases inflammation in blood vessels, increasing blood flow and arousal. Pumpkin seeds are a rich source of polyunsaturated fatty acids proven to boost prostaglandins that play a major part in libido.

- **Quinoa** – pronounced 'keenwa'. It is one of the few plant-based sources of complete protein available and not just found in health shops. It is also one of the top high-fibre foods. It takes a much longer time for the body digest fibre, so eating quinoa will provide your body with longer-lasting energy levels.

- **Red wine**. Yes, we shouldn't, but we do and what better excuse than

A clinical study showed that red wine can <u>increase the production</u> of male sex hormones testosterone. But interestingly too, it that is also one of the foods that can increase women's libido as well.

In another clinical study it was reported that it can <u>enhance the blood flow</u> toward a woman's erogenous zone. Som as well as boosting a woman's libido, it helps in lubrication, a solution for those experiencing vaginal dryness.

There is a relaxation benefit in that a glass of wine can also drive away stress and when we feel more restful, we're likely to have more energy and focus during sex.

- **Saffron** is a natural aphrodisiac, known for its ability to help improve sex drive in both men and women. It is well known to boost energy and improve stamina during love making.
In a clinical study on men with infertility issues, saffron was proven to <u>improve libido and erectile function</u>.

  Further evidence in another clinical study specifically on women with low sexual desire due to using antidepressants, saffron <u>was proven to improve lubrication and sexual desire</u>.

- **Spinach**. Those of a certain age cannot mention spinach without recalling Popeye but there is scientific evidence that Olive was wise to stick with Popeye for such a long time. Why was he obsessed with eating spinach? Surely it was ruse just to encourage kids to eat their veg. In fairness, back in the day we probably weren't aware that spinach has penis-enhancing power amidst its <u>high arginine content</u>. We're back to nitic acid again, when the amino acid hits in spinach gets into your system, it converts to nitric oxide, this helps initiate and maintain erections.

- **Tomato** is one of the foods that does increase libido in men, this is due to lycopene, a powerful antioxidant. It boosts prostate health too, this in turn improves virility in men.

- **Tuna** has a lot going for it. Containing vitamin B12 for quick energy boosts. It helps maintain healthy nerves, brain, and red blood cells. In a study published by Harvard University in the _New England Journal of Medicine_, lack of vitamin B12 isn't good for your sex life, promoting fatigue, low libido as well as erectile dysfunction, and weakness in the body. However, canned tuna is one of the top five sources of the micronutrient that helps.

- **Watermelon** is one of the richest natural sources of L-citrulline, a non-essential amino acid that your body converts to L-arginine in your body. L-citrulline is used in medicine for heart failure as well as for improving athletic performance and erectile dysfunction. It is the L-arginine that can help make an erection become harder, like the famous little blue pills. L-arginine stimulates the production of nitric oxide, and increases blood flow to the penis, strengthening erections. _Research published in the US National Library of Medicine_ Oral L-citrulline supplementation improves erection hardness in men with mild erectile dysfunction.

- **Wild salmon**. A great source of omega-3 fatty acids, which aid nitric oxide production as mentioned earlier and according to research published in the journal _Food & Function_, it helps with a longer lasting harder erection. A Mediterranean-style diet rich in produce, fish, whole grains, and healthy fats (like omega-3s) can improve erectile function, according to an _International Journal of Impotence Research_ study.

The vast majority of health advice anywhere is to eat as much fruit and vegetables as you can, drink plenty of water (2 litres per day, or 8 glasses is mainly suggested), and get as much sunlight as you feel you can safely handle.

Whilst the daily recommended servings of vitamins may t
a lot of nutritionists

recommends.

When you go the fridge for a 'glass' of orange juice, it is true that before you know it you have drank had half the carton in one go?
Our body can often crave stuff when we need more vitamins than we're receiving, and that craving can manifest itself into a binge just to absorb vitamins.

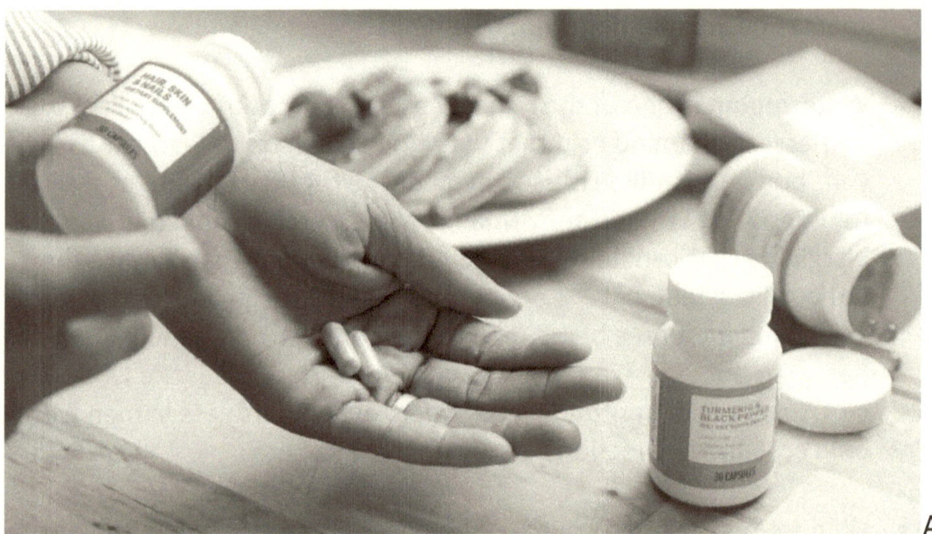

A lot of products claim to have 'added vitamins and minerals', including some bottled water.

Although, on the surface it may appear to be a good a way to help take on board plenty of your nutritional quota, but routinely getting an overload of vitamins and minerals can be harmful.

Did you know that:

- Overdoing vitamin C or zinc can cause nausea, diarrhea, and stomach cramps.

- Too much selenium can cause hair loss, stomach upset, tiredness, and mild nerve damage.

Sex in Your 60's

Most people don't really take a megadose, but if you aye say, a fortified cereal such as a simple bowl of cornflakes at breakfast, and grab an energy bar to see you between meal and then a bowl of enriched pasta for dinner, plus taking your daily supplement, you could well be going over the recommended daily intake of a host of nutrients.

There is no real advantage in taking more than the recommended amounts of vitamins and minerals, you don't gain anything positive, however there may be disadvantages to over doing it.

The best thing is to talk with your doctor about any vitamin supplements you are taking or intend to take, even though they are off the shelf vitamins and minerals. This approach ensures your doctor will help you keep doses in a safe range.

If you are taking a basic multivitamin supplement, there is no real need to be worried about taking too many because most multivitamins have a wide margin of safety that even when you're combining them with fortified foods, it is still won't cause you to go into trauma.

This isn't to say that they are harmless in overdose, in fact any ingredient in a multiple vitamin supplement can be toxic in large quantity, but the most serious risk comes from iron or calcium.

There is little or no evidence of anyone taking a toxic level of vitamin A or D for example, and it is very unusual, but if a person takes a dosing level of vitamin or mineral supplements that is higher than the stated recommended dose there may some signs that include sleeping difficulties, lack of concentrating, nerve problems such as numbness or tingling, feeling more irritable, but all these really depend on the nutrient that is going overboard.

Don't exceed the stated dose – simple!

Beat the Cravings

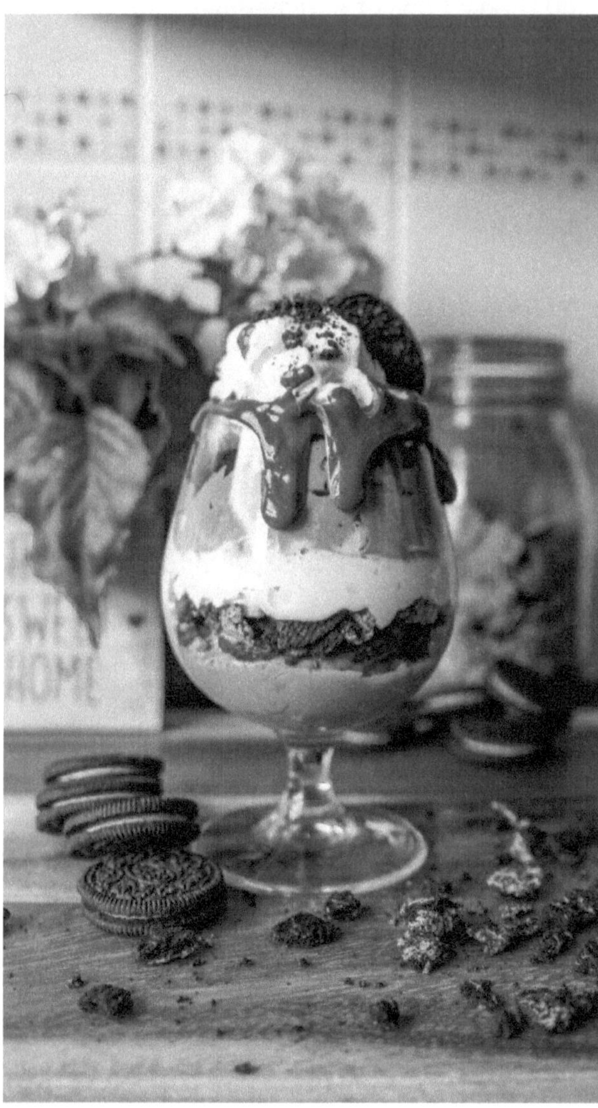

Craving can become a big issue especially after the end of a long relationship.

A person may find themselves feeling down or even going through depression, gaining weight and getting ill much more often than normal, despite still providing themselves with plenty of nutrition and exercise.

Nutrition, exercise and sex are three of the most incredibly useful tools to put towards maintaining a healthy, productive, active lifestyle, no matter what age you are.

But…. A little of what you fancy might make you feel better. So they say.

Just make sure your treat isn't going to be a punishment.

WANT TO BECOME A LOVE GOD OR GODDESS? (AGAIN)

Gone forever are the days of women being expected or demanded that the man to take charge or even initiate the encounter ask for a date, dance etc.

Today, a woman has the right including the responsibility to be equally

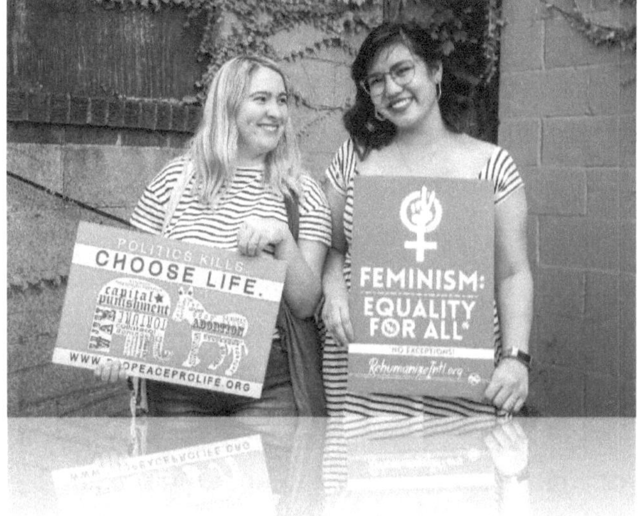

knowledgeable, giving, dedicated, and romantic as their partner.

It is now history for women to into marriages and expect their husband to lead them.

Today both the husband and wife are expected to enter their relationship equally but with openness and

willingness to learn and grow together as a couple.

If we were to be totally honest we would have to admit that it is extremely difficult reach the ages of fifty or sixty without picking up plenty of skills, but having said that, it equally not uncommon for a couple to be together for decades without ever learning more than one or two sexual positions or deeply exploring each other's preferences and indeed fantasies.

Be mindful now that new tricks are not really a powerful method of reinvigorating a romantic relationship that may be be viewed as a way of making the sex more fun than it has been previously.

Look at it as time to make sex new again, explored new territory, learn new things and don't be ashamed or embarrassed to suggest as well as try them.

Special new positions and toys are often recommended as a substitute for marriage guidance, counseling or even divorce, in the more extreme cases, remember, a strong sexual relationship really needs a strong personal relationship first and foremost.

There is a description often used for 'same old, same old sex', and that is 'vanilla'. A vast number of people that regularly indulge in sex without romantic attachments often declare that their sex was significantly more rewarding when carried out with a partner whose company is enjoyable outside of bed.

This means that they don't need sex to enjoy each other, they have fun together outside the bedroom too. There is no sexual technique that is truly magical, even more so, if your relationship is experiencing serious problems, good sex not going to fix it and the only responsible action is to try your best to work it out. That is not to say that truly good sex cannot be an excellent incentive to work things out, but, it takes much more than great love making skills to maintain a positive relationship.

A good way to do this is to start dating again, not with other partners but with each other. Go on fun dates, cinema, events, outings etc. Enjoy a meal out just like you did when you first dated.

Learn about each other's bodies again. Time has passed, senses have altered, shapes have changed. So, start again by exploring each other, softly, slowly and let your partner know what is nice, what is good, really good and wow!

There are so many things a person can try, and do, it is important to experiment. Look at one of the various books about sexual techniques and positions, these will help you achieve a more thorough modern education on the art of sex.

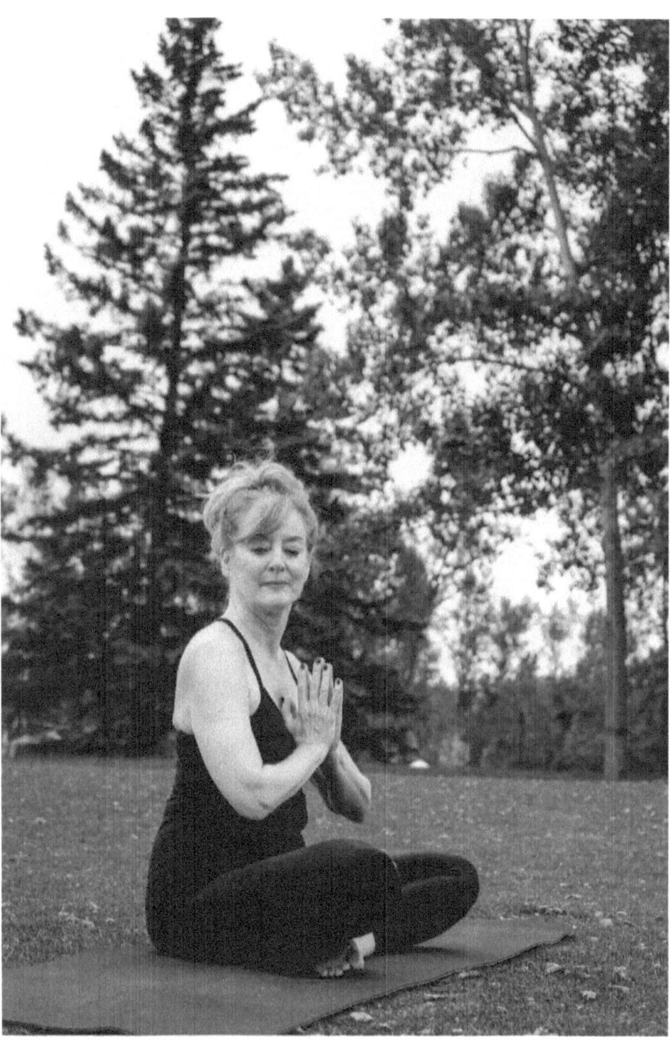

Whether you are over 50, 60 or even 70, our backs and knees can tend to get a bit creaky from time to time, also the pain can put us off from active sex.

So, experiment with positions that may have no discomfort or distractions and worrying if your partner is uncomfortable.

It really does makes sense to try and test some positions until you find a few that will feel as comfortable as possible.

The following part is just an introduction or a reminder course to hopefully encourage you to pursue your lovemaking further.

WOMEN ON TOP

There are quite a few positions for women to enjoy sex on top, some need good knees, other are fun instigating a session.

a lot men prefer to be on top of his female partner all of the time and far too often the female never gets the opportunity to try different positions.

Many men like to be on top, it could be said for selfish reasons because it is simply more physically fulfilling him. However, there are those men who just are not secure enough in their own self esteem to let their partner to have the dominant position.

Many women prefer the sexual experience when they are on top as they can adjust speed and rhythm, so the lovemaking becomes much more rewarding for them.

It is of course a personal choice, and if a female has never had the opportunity to try it, the very least a caring, unselfish man can offer his partner is the opportunity to try and see how she likes being on top and in charge.

- **Cowgirl.** Think about a rodeo, pink cowboy hat not essential but could be fun! The man on his back with the woman facing away from him and mounted him.

   This position is good for both partners, because women get deep penetration and can control speed, rhythm and her orgasm, it makes sensual contact with both the G-spot and the clitoris.

   The is also the benefit of appreciating each other visually, eye contact can really improve climax, and cowgirl position creates a tighter sensation which is pleasurable for both.

Cowgirl position is excellent for women who are going through menopause, because it helps intensify some of the sensations of sex.

It's easier on your lover's back too.

- **Reverse Cowgirl**

Women tend to enjoy reverse cowgirl, although some men with small penises may find it a little uncomfortable or unfulfilling, sometimes a tad awkward, or even impossible. However, if you feel it is worth trying, you may find it satisfactory to both partners, it does come highly recommended so don't dismiss the idea.

Once the woman is in position, she can lean forward, lean back, or sit upright, depending on personal preference.

- **Chest on chest**
It is what it says, but the difference here is this position simply involves the woman lying on her stomach on top of the man. Her legs are spread farther apart or held tight depending on personal choice. An excellent position if stamina is an issue, because it allows the woman to release pressure on the penis by spreading her legs, thus allowing for a longer encounter.

- **Chair position.**
An iconic photo is that of Christine Keeler straddled naked across a cheap office chair by photographer Lewis Morley. The chair position is the male sitting down and the woman straddles his lap, facing him, It is important to note that the chair needs to be low enough to the floor so that the woman can touch the ground with her feet to steady herself as well as give her leverage.

The best of two worlds is that this seated position is not only

If one partner has bad hips or has recently had hip-replacement surgery, give it a go!

MAN ON TOP

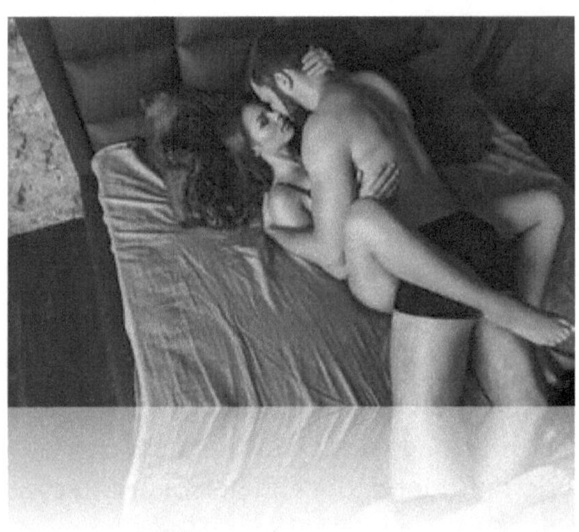

It is highly likely that you have already tried at least one of these positions and may be more simply because they are traditional positions where the man takes the dominant sexual position.

Forget the top position being reserved for the man, it may have been in the past, but no longer. The choice of being on top is so the person in that position really takes control of the situation, perhaps for greater pleasure, perhaps to see their partner, there is clearly the point that a man or indeed a woman will simply prefer to have pleasure given to them.

Rear entry, aka doggy style
This position has the woman on her hands and knees (hence 'doggy') with the man mounting her from behind. It is a position that is enjoyed by many couples because it has a number of benefits; the penis is naturally tilted slightly downwards so can rub up against the G-spot.

The female can also have control over the depth of penetration by lowering herself onto her elbows to increase it or reducing the arch in your back to decrease penetration.

The clitoris is in an ideal position to be stimulated by either party, alternatively the man can fondle her breasts and she can stimulate her own clitoris.

So, even if either suffer from bad knees, you will both be able to enjoy this position without too much discomfort.

- **Scissors**
  This is a popular position for the fact that it grants both partners some control. The position has the woman lie on her back and raise one leg, with the man straddling her lower leg and entering beneath her upper thigh. The woman can use her leg to control the tempo. This position is considered very intimate, allowing the lovers to hold one another and kiss.

- **Spread eagle**
  The woman lies on her stomach and spreads her legs as the man lies atop her. This position is more intimate than rear entry, allowing the man to kiss the woman or nibble on her ears, but can be uncomfortable for the woman when the man is heavier or has an unusually large penis.

- **Armchair**
  This position has the man and woman holding one another as in missionary, with the exception that the woman is sitting on an armchair, sofa, or bed, with the man kneeling before her. This allows both the man and the woman to better control the thrust of the love making as either partner can grip the arms of the chair for better stability.

Spooning is best-known for its cuddle position and for many, it's more of a

For the best effect, the male cuddles up to the female's back. She nudges her buttocks back, pressing against him and he can penetrate her from behind or lift her leg so he can enter her from an angle. In simple terms it is doggie style, but with no pressure on knees, a great position for those suffering from bad backs not to mention larger tummies.

Zen Pause.
With both partners lying on their backs, the female throws her nearest leg to the male over his body and finds an angle that allows entry. It is more of a side-by-side position and perfect for enjoying a close tender and relaxing moment with your partner. It's fun trying too

Doggy
Not the greatest of names but we all know what it is. A position where the female gets on her hands and knees making sure they are on a comfy surface, while the male kneels straight up behind and enters.

Ideal for deep penetration, it stimulates the G-spot, and can make it easier to reach around for manual stimulation.

Those who have recently had a hysterectomy and are easing back into sex after being cleared by a doctor will find this position works wonders.

Downward Facing
This position is ideal for those who have back pain although it might seem counterintuitive, this position helps because the male doesn't actually bend his back. Instead he holds steady on all fours and thrusts with his hips.

The female partner leans down on her elbows, often with her forehead to the mattress, and tilts her hips up.

This way, there is little or no strain on her neck and she places most of her weight on her arms and upper chest, rather than on her knees.

For men who have had prostate issues and not so hard erections, this may be a really good option because it creates a deeper and tighter sensation of penetration.

Stand up and from behind.
Many a spontaneous sex session has been instigated by that approach from behind. Standing up is not for everyone but for those it suits, it is a great way to boost your sex life and protect your joints too!

For this position, she leans forward with hands, elbows, or chest against a firm surface, it could be a kitchen worktop, back of the sofa, chair or even fireplace. he penetrates from behind.

There are challenges for couples who are not of equal height, but they can be creative.

The added bonus in this position is it can provide easy access for hand to clit stimulation, and no pressure on the shoulders, elbows, and hands.

FOREPLAY

Oral sex – Fellatio (On the man).
If you spoke with ten different people about their views on oral sex, you would get 15 different answers because a lot of them have mixed views.

Some women genuinely enjoy performing oral sex and there are men who when they find a woman who honestly enjoys performing oral sex, he's sorted and believes all else he needs in life is the simple bare necessities of life and he's in paradise.

Some women will have oral sex with their partner because she loves him, and he enjoys it. It also applies the other way around.

Some men expect oral sex but don't like reciprocating and that also works the other way around.

Some people, even in their 60's may never have had oral sex/fellatio. Or perhaps never had GOOD oral sex!

Good fellatio is powerful, it really cannot be overstated. Receiving meaningful oral sex, whether you are male, or female can be classed as the best part of sex.

It is even more satisfying for your partner if they know you are enjoying giving oral sex, so it is important before you even begin, to make sure that they know you enjoy doing it.

It is equally important for the receiver to make the right noises (literally) so that the giver knows there is proper enjoyment and what actions work in certain areas.

The act of oral sex doesn't need be performed in the dark, there's lots of positives about enjoying it in a well-lit room too.

The best place for oral attention is around the head of the penis and the part that connects the head of the penis to the shaft, the circumference of the base of the head. It is called the corona, the corona of glans penis or penis crown and is the most sensitive part of the penis.

The shaft itself isn't as sensitive as people would believe based on how the girls in X rated movies perform – don't be misled or disappointed that you are doing it wrong. Focus your attention on the end of the penis. Many men enjoy stimulation of the testicles at the same time.

The most important thing to remember about fellatio is don't hold back in really getting intimately familiar with your partner's penis.

Fully explore with your hands and mouth, you'll soon discover his sensual spots and remember, it may take several sessions before you become really good at it, and the reward is that your partner will worship you when you have got it right.

It's no secret that oral sex on a man is called a 'blow job', or 'giving head', or 'going down on him', and the best way to give a good blow job, or give good head is to use all parts of your mouth. If you think it is about sucking, you probably couldn't be further from the truth.

If you really want to excite his senses lick the whole length of his penis with the broad and flat part of your tongue, not just the tip. Making eye contact while you do this not only shows you are enjoying it, but it is an incredible turn on too.

The head or tip of his penis is the most sensitive area because it is where most of the nerve endings are, so pay some attention here but move around freely to ensure all parts of that penis is getting your attention

Sex in Your 60's

One of the aspects about a 'blow job' that put some givers off is the thought of going deep, commonly known as 'deep throat'. You will be pleased to know that you can avoid it without him missing out on that pleasure. Holding the base of his penis with your hand and move it up and down in time with your mouth, this action gives the sensation deep throat but without making it uncomfortable for you.

Blow jobs are not just about mouth action, your hands too can add extra pleasure. Try gently playing with his balls, run your fingertips all the way up his inner thighs, or reach up and pinch his nipples.

A word of warning about jaw ache! You may be using muscles around your mouth that you don't normally use, so don't be ashamed or worried about pausing for a break, use your hands, rub his penis on and around your nipples, come up for a kiss, touch yourself because it is about both of you having good sex.

No need to maintain a regular rhythm, it will make him come quicker if that's what you want to of you want to bring him close to climax but then let him simmer, as you judge him coming, stop that action and move to a different area, tease him!

For Value Added Turn-on (VAT) let your partner hear you making noises while you are going down on them. There is also a sexy trick that you can do in creating vibrations by humming a drawn-out 'mmmmmmmmm' with your lips on his penis. If you want to take this a bit further, try holding a small vibrator against your cheek while his penis is in your mouth.

You're in control, so take full advantage and as he gets closer to climaxing, he may thrust powerfully into your mouth or instinctively grip your head. It may be a turn off for you, so pull away and tell him to slow down so you can enjoy it too. If you enjoy his thrust and climax in your mouth, carry one as you were.

Try stimulating your man's perineum (located between his anus and balls) by gently massaging it whilst performing oral sex.

ORAL SEX – CUNNILINGUS (ON WOMEN)

People can have as much enjoyment giving oral sex as receiving it. It is genuinely rewarding giving oral sex when your lover is making you very aware that you are the best.

It has been said that "a lover is really only as good as their ability to deliver oral sex".

A lot of women will happily tell you that men are rubbish at giving oral sex. Whose fault is that?? If you asked your partner to scratch your back, you would direct them wouldn't you…"left a bit, right a tiny bit and just down, ahh bliss"

The same could have been said about receiving a message. You make noises and comment about how good it is – so what is stopping you commenting and directing where the pleasure is, and indeed there is nothing stopping the giver from listening to their lover's responses and deliver accordingly,

So where do you start? Firstly, practice makes perfect and secondly, it takes two and both should play a part to ensure that oral sex is good for both.

If for any reason, you haven't actually had any experience at performing oral sex on your partner, here's a quick guide to help you become an expert very quickly.

To gain expertise in the art of oral sex, you simply need to practice, and every time you practice whole experience will be more and more rewarding when both partners open to new ideas, ways and positions.

instead you are using your mouth. Your age certainly does not mean your life is limited, so treat these intimate sessions as if you have all the time in the world with your partner. Explore different positions and be mindful that it doesn't have to be up in the air for oral sex.

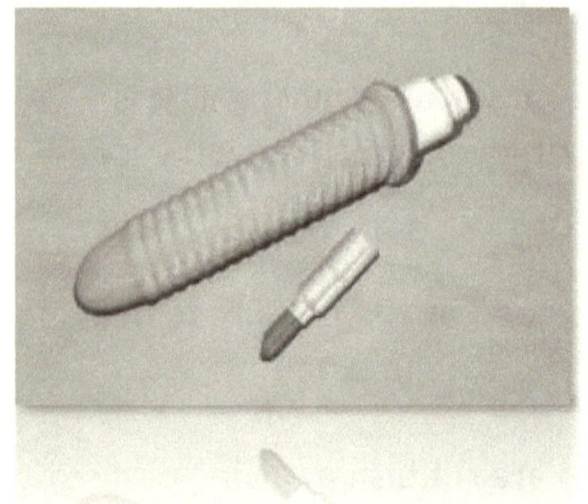

Toys are allowed too, Dildos, Vibrators and with consent, you might want to try a butt plug or anal beads for diversity, if you're not sure what they are, Google it!

Oral sex isn't just about licking and sucking, use your hot breath too, it will stimulate your partner's nerve endings is an amazing way.

As your mouth is approaching your partner's organ, slowly breathe on their sensitive parts before making contact. Remember, take your time, tease them with your breath because the suspense will turn them on in ways you, or they, didn't know existed.

Don't just go straight in and focus on the clitoris, spend time on her labia and everything else that deserves a vocal or physical response. So, if you are receiving, don't lay still and quiet… use your limbs and hips to let your partner know that whatever they are doing, it's good. Moan, talk, groan, tell them! Make sure you listen to your partner's signals too.

Your tongue isn't a stick or poker, relax it, use the tip, the sides, top and underneath of it, use your lips and a very gentle, soft touch with your hands,.

Men…. A word of advice, women is built differently to men as well as other women, they also think differently and as if you didn't know, they change their mind quite often. With this in mind, treat each and every time as if it's a new experience, never stop listening never stop trying new things. Most Women need more time to warm up than men do, so gentle touching is an excellent build up.

Some women's nipples seem to be directly wired to their clitoris, so don't neglect them, give them both plenty of attention and discover their lower exciting, turn on pain threshold by gently biting down or pinching them.

Work down to the vagina by kissing, licking and perhaps nibbling as you approach it.

It's a good thing to spread her labia (the inner and outer folds of the vulva (external part of the vagina), at either side of the vagina). during cunnilingus. A lot of people are quite shy about this, but in reality, you're both exposing your intimate parts, so, in for a penny, in for a pound and spread the labia wide, get into the folds, use your tongue to gently get into all the nooks and crannies, then the sensation will certainly improve.

Try sucking on her clitoris too, it delivers a very intense pressure. Some ladies enjoy a gentle flicking motion on their clitoris.

You can start with your fingers to open her vagina lips and use your thumbs to stroke gently, then move to using your tongue. Start by licking her with a very light touch then increase the pressure.

You can't take anything for granted when it comes to a woman's sensual areas so explore every fold, nook and cranny.

If you're moving upwards with your tongue, pout your bottom lip and let the inside of it follow your tongue, it's like being double licked.

Don't just lick up and down, women like is the "circular" motion that circles around the clitoris with a tongue too and for extra fun, spell yours or her name with your tongue, on her clit, for fun. Start with a light feathery action and build up the momentum, switch the motions between a more and a less intense touch. There is also the "dollar sign" and "side-to-side" lick. Inserting a finger or two when you feel she is getting aroused; you'll also know this because her breathing seems heavier and her thighs may tremble.

If you concentrate on her reactions, you will learn when

When she is about to come, use your tongue at this point in a very long up and down motion, engaging your lips too for double licking. Don't stop, keep repeating those licks. Listen for signs of escalating excitement, there include; deeper breathing, moaning, grunting, or even talking to their creator! Keep that up until her body tenses up and she lets it go. When do you stop? When she pushes you away or moves away, it's her call!

Try different positions, not just with her lying on her back. Some positions are better than others, depending on you both and how daring you are to try. Try it with her on all fours so you can give her your oral delights from behind. Try it with her standing and you are on your knees. (use on a pillow or cushion to protect your knees).

LUBRICATION

Quite often a woman reaches a timer in her life when her vagina doesn't naturally lubricate, usually at the menopause stage, and particularly if she is not using hormonal supplements.

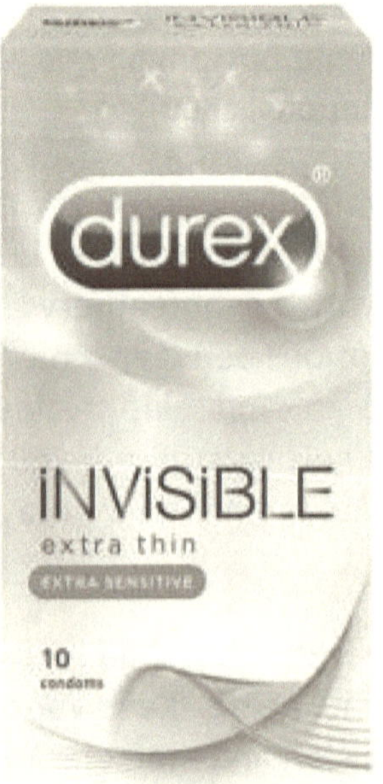

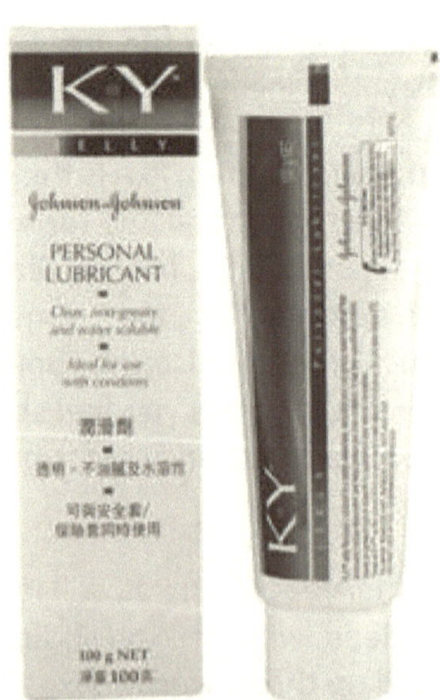

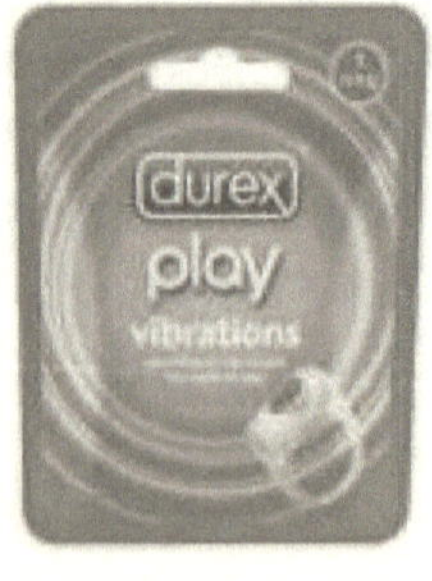

Sex in Your 60's

So, when a man was once prepared with condoms, now it is worth being prepared for If she is feeling dry, then lubrication is very handy. K-Y Jelly® for instance is easily available from grocers as well as pharmacies, or if you are shy, you can buy it online but despite the fact that it is intended to be used prior to or during intercourse to help minimize the discomfort that can occur due to vaginal dryness, if has 101 other uses such as:

Remove too-tight rings.
Open (or close) a stuck zipper.
Unstick a screw or bolt that won't loosen.
Remove goo residue from stickers.
Act as moisturizer.
Hair gel.
Remove gum from furniture.
Use as shave gel.
Heal severely cracked lips.
Shine your patent leather.

So, you don't need to be worried about being judged when you buy a tube of lube or two!

lubrication isn't just to make entry a lot smoother.

If you are feeling adventurous, you can buy flavoured lubricants to introduce more fun and games. In addition to flavoured options, there are lubes that is a choice of super-slippery water-based lubes, silicone lube, organic lubricant and anal sex lubrication.

Another option is Durex Play which lubricates and enhances orgasm.

It is important to make sure that foreplay is long and arousing to encourage natural lubrication, so men...be patient, take your time and concentrate on pleasing your partner.

if you start by caressing her over her knickers or stockings and use a bit of lube on your fingers, feels amazing for her.

ALL SEXES ARE EQUAL

The world is changing with regards to sex relationships in general between men and women, be in no doubt that men should expect their female sex partners to be assertive and voice
their needs.

Any man that wants to provide his partner with a satisfying sexual experience, he simply needs to listen to her, pay very close attention to what she says and what she does, and ask her questions if necessary.

You can read the most thorough, explicit book on sexual advice, but it will never equal the effectiveness of being a good listener and being attentive.

Of course, if you are over fifty or sixty and have been married to the same partner for many years, you would, we hope, know her and shouldn't need to be told about the importance of listening to women, but that importance is crucial and cannot be overemphasized.

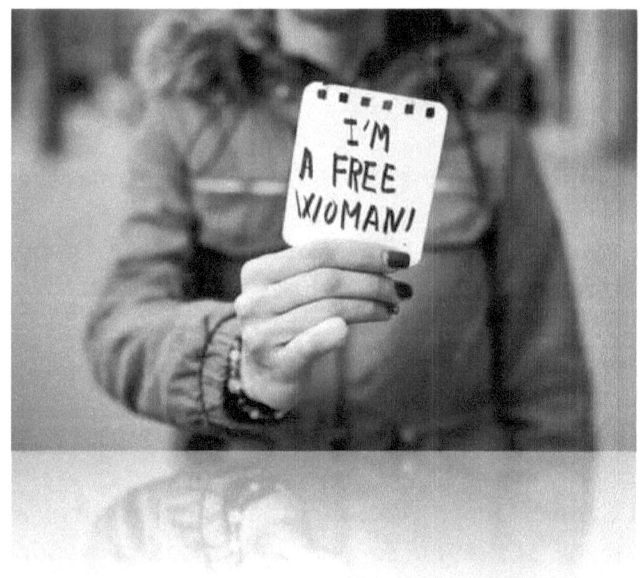

Be mindful that a man should expect to have
to discuss with his
partner her own preferences and dislikes well before he can ever consider himself a master of the art of making love.

Sex in Your 60's

If you are an attentive lover and have always been willing to be open minded and explore new things yet you are looking to improve your sex life with new tricks and perhaps surprise your wife of many years with your new wealth of sexual knowledge, you might need a library fool of volumes dedicated entirely to sexual techniques and positions, because this one that you are reading right now is but starter. However, it will serve you well as an introduction to better sex for those in their 50's and beyond. It might also provide some new ideas for the seasoned expert in love making.

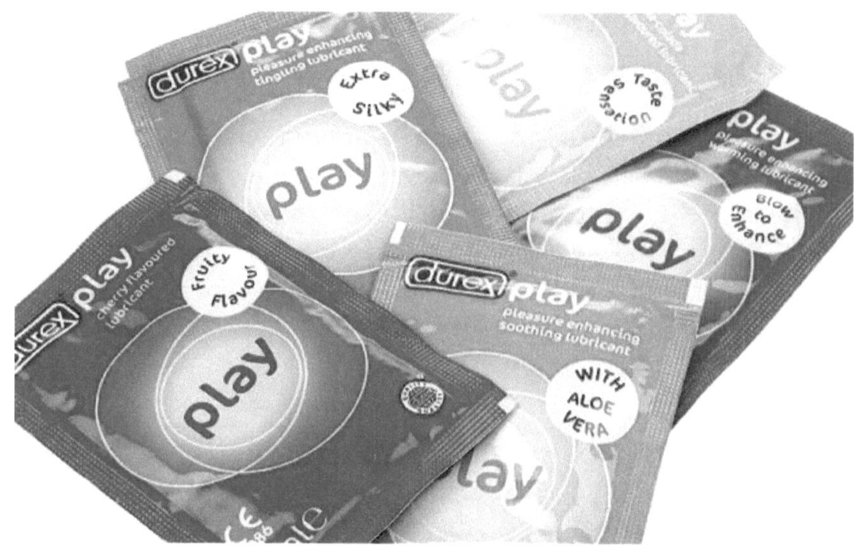

In truth, there are only so many variations of things we can do in bed. Newfangled sexual techniques alone will never provide the foundations of a serious relationship, and as much as tremendous sex will, without doubt strengthen a relationship, it can never save a failing one. All too often, sexual advice is given as some form of substitute for proper relationship advice, so be mindful that the tips here should be taken in the knowledge that, as important as sex is, serious problems must be worked through with guidance from a professional counselor, not the help of a sex book.

LOVE YOURSELF

Perhaps when you were in your 30's you thought anyone in their 60's was very, very old. When you got into your 40's those 60-year old's didn't seem too old, and when your you're in your 50's and 60's, it really isn't that old.

Any fans of Full Metal Jacket or more recent 'Breaking Bad' may be aware of actor, R. Lee Ermey. If you searched Google for information about him, you would discover that he openly discussed his own masturbation habits.

During a recent interview, a topic came up about the art of leaving something to the imagination, it is quoted that he said "If you have an imagination anywhere near what mine is like, I mean, I still masturbate for Christ's Sakes! I can still visualize Marilyn Monroe and the Playboy bunnies from the 1950s". So, if anybody had any doubt as to when men stop masturbating, it is certainly not in their 60's!!

MASTURBATION MAY BE GOOD FOR YOU

https://www.independent.co.uk/life-style/health-and-families/health-news/masturbation-can-be-good-for-the-over-50s-1516792.html

The UK's Independent Newspaper

Masturbation can be good for the over 50's

Masturbation has been proven time and time again to have a host of benefits to a person's health. When men ejaculation they experience heightened arousal and this helps release epinephrine, a hormone cited by many professionals as helping to relieve depression and stress.

Ejaculation also helps to prevent prostate cancer.

Marc Garnick, M.D., Editor in Chief of Harvard Medical School's Annual Report on Prostate Diseases, *says:*

Two relatively large studies of this question, reported in 2003 and 2004, yielded good news for sexually active men: high ejaculation frequency seemed to protect against prostate cancer.

https://www.health.harvard.edu/blog/does-frequent-ejaculation-help-ward-off-prostate-cancer-20090929112

Whatever one's feelings are on masturbation, everybody does it, with the odd few exceptions. Those who don't indulge tend to have suffered a form of sexual trauma in the past or possibly brought up with a very negative view of sex generally.

Masturbation is not a sign of perversion but rather, a sign of a healthy sexual appetite and not necessarily for those alone, it it also practiced by those in sexually active relationships. It isn't a substitute for sex, but more like enjoying sex with one's self. People play games by themselves, go for walks by themselves, go to the cinema by themselves. Masturbation is also accepted as a compromise in maintaining the balance in a sexual relationship where one partner has a higher interest in sex than the other and is not judged for masturbating to meet their personal needs.

Mutual masturbation is more common than many would believe, it is indeed an intimate form of sexual intercourse, involving a couple using their hands to stimulate one another rather than indulging in penetration.

It may be that the main reason for masturbation is simply to satisfy sexual needs during times of being single bearing in mind that many individuals over 60 find themselves in the unfortunate position of being widowed or recently divorced or otherwise living on their own for the first time in years.

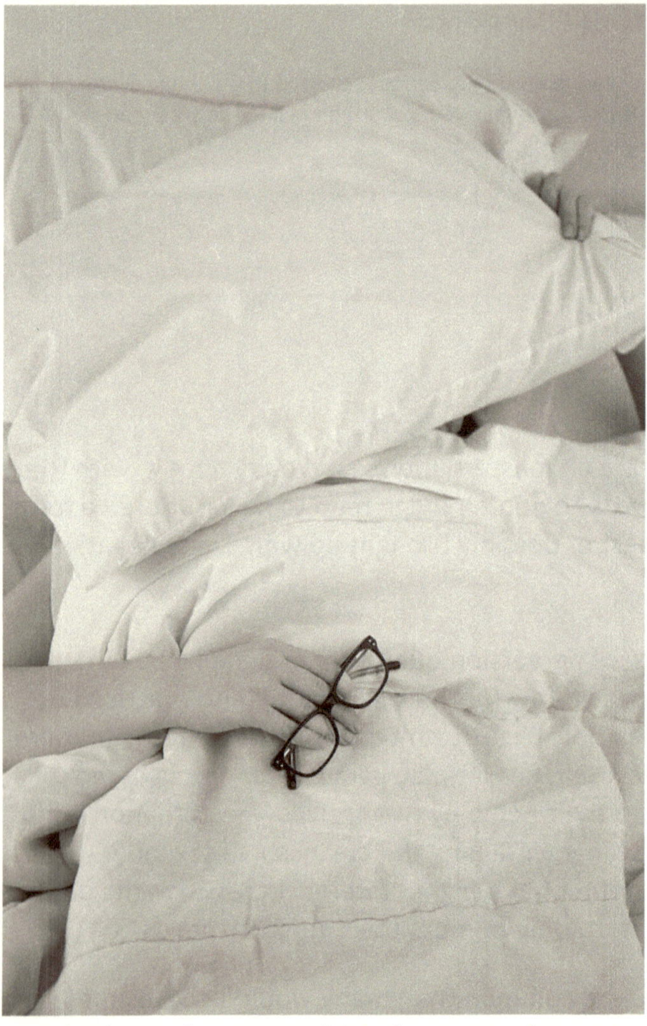

Being single at the age of over sixty is no reason to become a recluse and/or giving up on ever finding another sex partner.

Women can also enjoy the use of sex toys as well as hand masturbation, but these toys provide additional experiences during sexual intercourse.

It is true that some men can be very insecure if such toys are larger than their own penis, also men may feel this activity is outside their own comfort zone.

The good news is that you don't need to surreptitiously venture into a sex product shop, they can be bought discreetly online.

DON'T Let a Medical Condition HOLD You Down

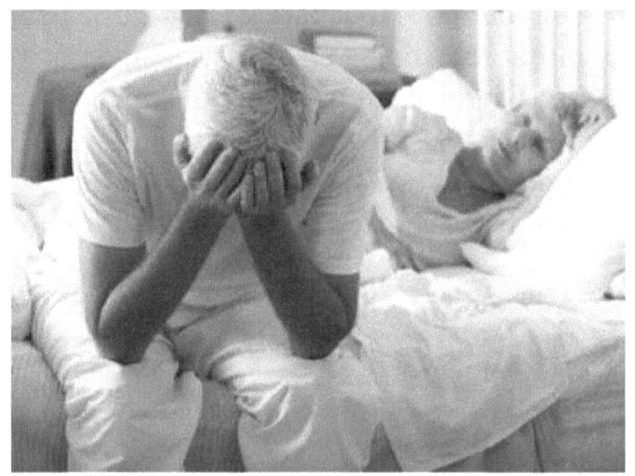

Life is a lottery and no matter how well we take care of ourselves, no matter how strict we are on healthy eating, and how regular we, health will deteriorate as we live longer and some of us will still be healthier than others despite the condition of our health.

As time moves on, we need to make some changes in our lifestyle, it may be a simple things like acquiring a hearing aid or needing to take regular medication, but sadly some of us will suffer major life-changing conditions causing limitations in our basic abilities.

It's not all about how we live our life to stay healthy, Some illnesses are hereditary, there are the cases of unfortunate accident, falling victim by being in the wrong place at the wrong time and the added irony of being involved in an accident whilst on a keep fit activity.

Ultimately we hope that no matter what condition your health is, we hope you still have the desire to live an active sex life and there is no reason to give up on sex.

If you are unfortunate enough to be in a condition where you need to adjust in order to still enjoy a sexual relationship with your partner it it important that you share your concerns and fears so you both can work together and find ways to still enjoy sex.

potential partner about your health conditions and concerns. This isn't to say you should meet and greet a potential sex partner and before you have even sat down, you confess that sex might be a problem!

Remember, it is nothing to be embarrassed about. Yes, it can be difficult to build the courage to talk about it, but your potential partner is likely to be delighted that you did bring it up, rather than being embarrassed and compromised. it may be that they too would like to chat about concerns they have, so ultimately you will find yourselves involved in a sincere discussion about the changes your body has gone through in recent years, far less an embarrassing chat than you first expected.

WHAT CAN POSSIBLY GO WRONG?

Here's some tips on how to deal with common health problems that may affect one's sex life. It is important note that these topics and any major conditions that have not yet been mentioned here must be discussed in depth with a doctor as well as with one's sexual partner.

- **Erectile dysfunction**
  Viagra often come to mind when people think about erectile dysfunction but before you head off to the doctor for a Viagra prescription, be mindful that erectile dysfunction isn't exclusive to men over sixty. Young men even those only just out of their teen years can suffer from erectile dysfunction. This condition can be as a result of a deficiency in vitamins and other vital nutrients. So, before focusing on Viagra, why not try a change in diet and exercise habits first?

- **Diabetes**
  Erectile dysfunction can also be evident with those suffering from Diabetes. High blood sugars can be the cause of blood vessel and

nerve issues which may affect sexual responsiveness. There's also high cholesterol that can slow blood flow due to fatty deposits. On a positive note, improving the quality of one's sex life can in turn be very good incentive to monitor one's blood sugar levels.

- **Loss of bladder control**
  Earlier in this publication Kegel exercises were mentioned. Loss of bladder control can be embarrassing but easily remedied. To strengthening bladder control, do some with Kegel exercises! Of course, an obvious solution is simply to drink too much before sex.

- **Menopause and andropause**
  We don't hear much about andropause – it is a condition of decreasing testosterone in men that usually begins to occur at about 40 years of age. However, Menopause and andropause can result in a reduced sex drive. Yet again, something that can sometimes be fixed with a change in diet, however, it is likely that some medical attention will be required. There are pills and injections readily available by prescription that can help to improve your hormone levels.

Cancer

There are a number of cancer types including; testicular cancer, prostate cancer, cervical cancer and breast cancer, all of which can negatively affect a person's sex life. It is worth noting that when a cancer survivor is fortunate enough to come out the other end of that long dark tunnel with no immediate issues in a physical sense, that will affect their sexual ability, however there is emotional trauma of losing a breast or a testicle that can be devastating and could damage one's self esteem, this can lead to a loss of interest in sex and worse still, can result in complete inability to perform.

forth and enjoy sex!. Keeping on top of it (pun intended) is important and women should regularly carry out self-checks and obviously consult their doctor about any unusual abdominal cramps or aches. Foreplay is a great way to check one another for cancer. Don't feel like you are scaremongering if you bring to your partner's attention any abnormalities in their body, it is important that it is brought to their immediate attention so they can see their doctor.

Self-esteem can naturally suffer after invasive surgery or indeed amputation, let's face it, it is very difficult to look into a mirror and see a body that is no longer what you are used to seeing. What is important is to understand that you are no less of a person than you were before. Seriously consider joining a support group that fits your needs or a seek a therapist that is well equipped to help cancer survivors, there are plenty of cancer charities that can assist in finding the right people to help.

Ladies (and men) who have lost a breast to cancer and chose not to have a breast implant may opt to have a tattoo in place of a breast. There's a lot of scares due to news about health problems associated with breast implants (a high number of men too). The tattoo option has become quite a trend and good example of an empowerment, an excellent method in exerting control over the appearance of one's own body.

So in summary about cancer, it should not destroy your sex life. Reclaim it right now and get a sign that says 'business as usual', put it above your bed! – on second thoughts it might send the wrong message to anyone who sees it, but you get the idea. The 'business as usual' attitude is a very powerful life-affirming way to deal with that emotional trauma after invasive surgery.

BEYOND THE BLUE PILL

Put aside all the cheap jokes about Viagra (sildenafil citrate), funny or not, let's take Viagra seriously because there is no doubt that the blue pill has been an invaluable help to thousands upon thousands of men over the age of sixty.

Men can now buy Viagra Connect without a prescription at some UK pharmacies.

To obtain Viagra Connect in the UK you simply need to have a short conversation with the pharmacist. Restrictions are generally that men who become very breathless or experience chest pain when doing light exercise, such as climbing two flights of stairs, should not take these pills.

A packet of four pills will cost £19.99 (British Pounds)

The generic version of Viagra, sildenafil, is now available in the United States. Compare prices among local pharmacies and Canadian or international online pharmacies by using this link. Paying cash may be cheaper than using insurance.

Don't be ashamed of having erectile dysfunction. It is better to see a doctor now that spending your next 30 or 40 years being frustrated and lonely.

Remember earlier in this publication we covered poor diet and an inactive lifestyle; these are at the core of just about every common health problem. If you can simply eat a little more in the way of fresh fruit and vegetables as well as grains and if you smoke, cutting back or stop'. Even reducing your caffeine intake and alcohol could solve your problems without the need for medications.

There are always exceptions to the rule of diet and exerci
cases, it is impossible to convi

they would feel much better if they went for walk around the block each morning.

Usually when someone feels fatigued, lacks energy, suffers from erectile dysfunction, lacks interest in most things and feels low, all add up to sexual hang-ups and could well be related to the lack of a proper diet and activity. It becomes a vicious circle. Having said that, someone feeling those symptoms may be put off decent healthy food, so we can't blame the diet but it becomes part of the problem.

Below are some issues that you may experience (hopefully you don't), but may need to seek medical advice to improve your sex life, it is just a brief list of what you could discuss with your partner or doctor about as potential means for treatment.

A comprehensive list of every single one of the many and various causes of decreased libido would certainly fill a one thousand page encyclopedia, so this chapter is limited and unfortunately cannot list them all

- **Erectile dysfunction**

Viagra is the most common brand, alternatives are:
  - **Vardenafil:** Sold under the brand names Levitra and Staxyn
  - **Tadalafil:** Available under the brand names Adcirca and Cialis
  - **Avanafil:** Marketed in the U.S. as Stendra

They are called PDE5 inhibitors very efficient ways to deal with erectile dysfunction.

There are non-oral drugs for erectile dysfunction, some of which can be considered as very inconvenient and unpleasant

- **Penile self-injections:**

Medications such as alprostadil, papaverine, and phentolamine, can be injected directly into the side or base of the penis (ouch!). These injections help to achieve or maintain an erection for up to 40 minutes.

- **Urethral suppository:**

Another 'ouch' because tiny alprostadil suppositories are placed down the urethra using a specially designed applicator. An erection occurs within 10 minutes and can last for up to an hour.

- **Testosterone replacement:**

If a man is suffering from low levels of testosterone, a doctor may suggest this treatment it can be delivered by a choice of routes, including injection, patch, or oral medication.

With the introduction and ease of access to Viagra, a lot of these are outdated or least preferred for obvious reasons.

However, before you commit to taking 'the little blue pill', consider talking with a therapist as it really can help, and is often recommended to be tried before considering Viagra. If erectile dysfunction is the result of a psychological issue, discussing that issue with a therapist may assist in aiding the process of dealing with erectile dysfunction. If the cause is not psychological, a therapist might help to discount any subconscious hang-ups, as well as with any distress that may be as a direct result of the erectile dysfunction.

- **Decreased libido**

Don't blame 'old age' if you're 'off sex'. Far too many people simply cannot even be bothered do anything about their own libido when it on that slippery slope down. However, you, the reader are not one of those people who cannot be bothered, otherwise you wouldn't be reading this publication based on the fact that it is entirely focused on subject of sex after the age of sixty. However, alongside erectile dysfunction, a lack of interest in any kind of sex could well be attributed to psychological trauma that was suffered in life. It may even be the pure stress due to aging is enough to bring this lack of interest on. Think about this first, then examine

- **Sleep apnea**

Did you even imagine that sleep apnea or snoring could be a cause? It really is worth considering it as a candidate, especially if you have already ruled out psychological hang-ups. What is sleep apnea? It is a condition where a person suddenly stops breathing for as much as ten to thirty seconds at a time whilst they are sleeping. The US Library of Medicine reported that Men with untreated OSA (Obstructed Sleep Apnea) suffered from a low libido. Older age and depressed mood were the most important factors of low libido in middle-aged men with OSA.
https://www.ncbi.nlm.nih.gov/pubmed/30340202

Treatment is quite simple and straight forward. Doctors will generally prescribe a mouthpiece to wear whilst asleep, it retains the lower jaw in such a position as to open the airway, allowing for easier breathing. It might sound a tad awkward and clumsy, but the end result is increased energy and a good night's sleep.

- **Arthritis**

Another one that some people may question but those who have suffered from serious arthritis will testify just how bad it really is in terms of limiting their lifestyle choices. However, it is one of the easiest to treat, in most cases. Those that suffer with minor arthritis, may benefit from pain relievers and physical therapy for better mobility and comfort in bed. Unfortunately, sufferers of more intense arthritis might have to investigate other measures such as extreme surgery to replace broken joints. Rest and keeping fit with low impact exercise are pretty much all that is required, no matter how serious or minor the arthritis.

Whatever your situation, it is important that you confront whatever is standing between you and a healthy sex life, never give up on living your life exactly as you see fit.

Involving your Doctor

If you have a very young, newly qualified doctor, they may be totally open to listening to your problems and even welcome the idea of researching for solutions to help improve your sex-life. If however you a very young, newly qualified doctor that believes those over 60 should not be indulging in sex at their age, you may have a problem. There is an unfortunate presumption that people over sixty should grow old gracefully.

You may have a doctor who is old enough to understand that retiring doesn't mean an end to your sex life, or simply experienced enough not to be so narrow minded.

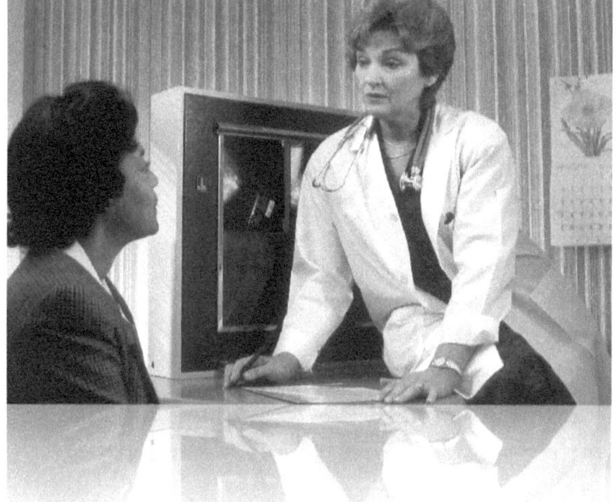

How, do you broach the subject about your sex life

You may be totally honest and up-front, have no hang-ups or concerns about discussing your sex life and you are happy to talk to your doctor about and even discuss preventative measures and proper lifestyle habits etc. Is your doctor going to be comfortable talking to you about sex though? There shouldn't be any reason why not if you ensure the dialogue is open and uninhibited. There really should be no taboo questions when it comes to your health, and your sex life is connected to your health.

It is crucially important that you seek a second opinion whenever the first opinion comes from a doctor who shows even the slightest signs disinterested. On that same note it may also be the best time to register with a new doctor if yours present one you with such disinterest. Afterall this is your health we're talking about.

Loss of libido

A couple of very simple questions to ask your doctor in relation to loss of libido. (loss of interest in sex)

- **"Could loss of libido have anything to do with the medication I am on?"**
Many medications do inhibit the libido, and it may be that you are not actually taking any that do affect your sex life on their own, it could be that two or three working together in your body can create such an effect.

- **"Could it be my lifestyle that is to blame?"**
Apart from the obvious diet and exercise issue, loss in libido can also be caused by excessive stress in your daily life or simply an underwhelming, disappointing day to day routine. Your hormone levels rely quite heavily on your emotions and it is crucially important to take care of yourself in all areas of your daily life if you want enjoy a fulfilling and healthy sexual appetite.

Don't be afraid to ask more general questions, you really do need to communicate with your doctor and be as direct as you possibly can. By giving him or her as much information as you possibly can, you are likely to get the most precise answers.

Pain During Sex

If you are experiencing some degree of pain during sex, it isn't unusual and has a broad range of causes, so when discussing this issue with your doctor, be as specific as possible. Your doctor needs to know where the pain, the type of pain and how it feels. If it is inside the opening of your vagina or inside the tip of your penis and is a stinging or throbbing pain for example.

Sex in Your 60's

No matter how embarrassed you are about engaging in such explicit detail, it needs to be treated, when it comes to your health and wellbeing, there is absolutely no reason to be ashamed or embarrassed.

Vaginal pain is not uncommon and generally caused by dryness, occurring often when there is little or no time for foreplay allowing the woman to become sufficiently aroused before penetration. It can usually be treated without a doctor's intervention as long as the woman is obviously willing to discuss the problem with her partner and strongly suggest, or even insist that they dedicate more time to foreplay during sex including the possible use of lubrication. Another issue may be lowered estrogen levels. More foreplay may solve this problem, if not, your doctor may prescribe hormones supplements.

A man experiencing pain in his genitals during sex, may be any number of problems and immediate consultation is of paramount importance. Soreness during or after sex may be something relatively minor such as eczema, fungal issue, or simply dryness (if this is the case, just drink more fluids and/or see your doctor). Do not dismiss the fact that it could relate to more serious problems. Minor aches and pains in the penis and especially relating to the testicles should be diagnosed as soon as possible.

It isn't just intimate pain that can cause problems during sex it can be due to arthritis for example. Since the act of sex actually exercises some parts of our body in ways that are almost exclusive to sexual activity, it isn't uncommon someone to realise they suffer from arthritis until they have sex. Over the counter medication may eliminate this type of pain, however, it should nonetheless be discussed with your doctor, as minor aches and pains could well be indicative of developing problems that may escalate in the fullness of time

BEING CAREFUL in the Twenty First Century - STD

Ok, you're over a certain age and perhaps it seemed like yesterday when you were advised to be careful or indeed, you were dishing out that same advice. STD's (Sexually transmitted diseases) are spread due to the exchange of bodily fluids and during sex there are quite a few of those including vaginal fluids, semen, pre-ejaculate, and blood.

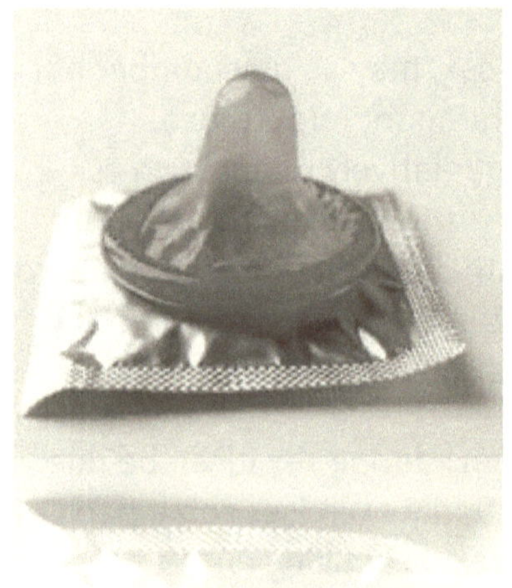

If you have just met a new sexual partner, you may feel you know them well and indeed met their family, learned of previous lovers and gained a bigger picture of their background. You may even feel confident that because their previous relationship was with just one partner for the last 25 years, so the risk of STD's is minimal.

Without interviewing their partner, you do not know if they had a very active sex life and had STD potentially passing it on to your new partner, who in turn could pass it on to you. It is always a good idea before having unprotected sex to get blood tests for both yourself and your new partner. Needless to say that sexual contact should really be avoided if you or your new partner have any angry spots, boils, open wounds or indeed are unsure of your own sexual health.

For a good idea of USA statistics for STDs click here.

Sex in Your 60's

Over 1 million STDs are acquired every day worldwide
There are an estimated 376 million new infections each year with
STDs:
Chlamydia
Gonorrhoea
Syphilis
Trichomoniasis

The World Health Organisation published and in-depth report on STD's –
click here.

A report of patients on athenahealth's network found that people age 60+
account for the biggest increase in treatments STDs. The report found that in
adults aged 60+ the diagnosis rates for herpes simplex, gonorrhea, syphilis,
hepatitis B, trichomoniasis and chlamydia rose by 23 percent between 2014
and 2017.

To see the 2018 report by the Centers for Disease Control and Prevention
click here.

One of the reasons why some women over 60 are opting for unprotected
sex is menopause. To pinpoint this further it is because the manner in
which some women behave following menopause. They may have
practiced safe sex all of their lives, mainly to avoid getting pregnant and
then chose to stop using condoms after menopause, in the safe knowledge
that they can no longer have children so there is no need to use
contraceptives.

In Summary

Continue to enjoy sex for as long as you want to do it – Remember the
saying, 'use it or lose it' and this is true whether it is with partner sex or
pleasuring yourself.